M000276088

SPIRITUALITY AND HOSPICE SOCIAL WORK

END-OF-LIFE CARE: A SERIES

END-OF-LIFE CARE: A SERIES

SERIES EDITOR: KEITH ANDERSON

We all confront end-of-life issues. As people live longer and suffer from more chronic illnesses, all of us face difficult decisions about death, dying, and terminal care. This series aspires to articulate the issues surrounding end-of-life care in the twenty-first century. It will be a resource for practitioners and scholars who seek information about advance directives, hospice, palliative care, bereavement, and other death-related topics. The interdisciplinary approach makes the series invaluable for social workers, physicians, nurses, attorneys, and pastoral counselors.

The press seeks manuscripts that reflect the interdisciplinary, biopsychosocial essence of end-of-life care. We welcome manuscripts that address specific topics on ethical dilemmas in end-of-life care, death, and dying among marginalized groups; palliative care; spirituality; and end-of-life care in special medical areas, such as oncology, AIDS, diabetes, and transplantation. While writers should integrate theory and practice, the series is open to diverse methodologies and perspectives. Manuscript submissions should be sent to series editor Keith Anderson at Keith.Anderson@mso.umt.edu.

Joan Berzoff and Phyllis R. Silverman, eds., *Living with Dying: A Handbook for End-of-Life Healthcare Practitioners*

Virginia E. Richardson and Amanda S. Barusch, *Gerontological Practice for the Twenty-first Century: A Social Work Perspective*

Ruth E. Ray, *Endnotes: An Intimate Look at the End of Life*

Terry Wolfer and Vicki Runnion, *Dying, Death, and Bereavement in Social Work Practice: Decision Cases for Advanced Practice*

Mercedes Bern-Klug, ed., *Transforming Palliative Care in Nursing Homes: The Social Work Role*

Dona J. Reese, *Hospice Social Work*

Allan Kellehear, *The Inner Life of the Dying Person*

Monika Renz, *Dying: A Transition*

Spirituality and Hospice Social Work

Ann M. Callahan

COLUMBIA UNIVERSITY PRESS   NEW YORK

COLUMBIA UNIVERSITY PRESS
Publishers Since 1893
New York   Chichester, West Sussex

cup.columbia.edu
Copyright © 2017 Columbia University Press
All rights reserved

Library of Congress Cataloging-in-Publication Data
Names: Callahan, Ann, author.
Title: Spirituality and hospice social work / Ann Callahan.
Other titles: End-of-life care.
Description: New York : Columbia University Press, [2017] |
    Series: End-of-life care | Includes bibliographical references and index.
Identifiers: LCCN 2016019911 (print) | LCCN 2016020785 (ebook) |
    ISBN 9780231171724 (cloth : alk. paper) | ISBN 9780231171731
    (pbk. : alk. paper) | ISBN 9780231543187 (e-book)
Subjects: | MESH: Hospice Care | Terminal Care | Spirituality
Classification: LCC R726.8 (print) | LCC R726.8 (ebook) | NLM WB 310 |
    DDC 616.02/9—dc23
LC record available at https://lccn.loc.gov/2016019911

Columbia University Press books are printed on permanent
and durable acid-free paper.
Printed in the United States of America

Cover design: Diane Luger

THIS BOOK IS DEDICATED TO MY GRANDMOTHER,
MARIE G. MERCIER, AND MY SPOUSE, TONI L. MCDANIEL.
THANK YOU FOR INSPIRING MY WORK AND HELPING ME
TO SUSTAIN IT.

CONTENTS

*SPIRITUALITY AND
HOSPICE SOCIAL WORK*

THE DYING PROCESS MAY BE considered a stage of life that is unique to each person. The process of dying is shaped by a collective of biopsychosocial and spiritual factors that change over time (Hospice Foundation of America, 2005; Lamers, 2014; Nuland, 1995; Reese, 2013). For example, the dying process may be shaped by the illness a patient has or the effect of medication (Lamers, 2014). The dying process may be shaped by the resources a patient has to cope with the challenges that living with dying creates. Within this fluid, subjective process of dying there can be growth and fulfillment (Reese, 2013). When this process is considered meaningful, it has been described as "dying well" (Byock, 1996). Spirituality may be one of those unique qualities that can make the end of life more meaningful. For some hospice patients, the meeting of spiritual needs is "an integral developmental task" (Puchalski, 2001, p. 353; see also Doka, 2011; Gijsberts et al., 2011; Hodge & Horvath, 2011; Penman, Oliver, & Harrington, 2013; Peteet & Balboni, 2013; Reese, 2013). Spiritual needs can lead to spiritual resilience or spiritual suffering, both of which may involve spiritual care. Therefore, it is important to understand the evolving nature of the dying process and how spirituality shapes this experience.

Research suggests that 80 to 90 percent of hospice-care patients may have spiritual needs (Gijsberts et al., 2011; Peteet & Balboni, 2013). Spiritual needs are described as a reflection of what a person values and what gives meaning to his or her life, which involves spiritual seeking or spiritual struggle (Glasper, 2011; Peteet & Balboni, 2013). The dying process can lead to feelings of loss, hopelessness, and abandonment, as well as forgiveness, peace, and acceptance, all of which can have spiritual implications (Hills, Pace, Cameron, & Shott, 2005; Lukoff, n.d.). Hospice social workers can identify a patient's spiritual needs and facilitate patient access to spiritual resources (Langegard & Ahlberg, 2009; Peteet & Balboni, 2013). However, spiritual needs are complex, and so is the process of addressing them. In response, hospice social workers need to be spiritually sensitive to recognize when it is necessary to facilitate spiritual care or build the spiritual competence to provide it (Edwards, Pang, Shiu, & Chan, 2010; Glasper, 2011). Educators and supervisors need this capacity, too, in order to train and support current and future hospice social workers. This book is intended to help by providing a review of key research that informs spiritually sensitive hospice social work. In this way, the experience of relational spirituality is possible through the provision of hospice social work.

NEED FOR TIMELY CARE

Hospice care has increasingly been an important resource for patients nearing the end of life. According to the National Hospice and Palliative Care Organization (NHPCO, 2014, 2015a), there has been steady growth in the number of hospice providers and patients served over the past decade. Between 2009 and 2014, the number of hospice patients increased from an estimated 1.3 million to 1.7 million. In 2014, 2.6 million people died in the United States, and 1.1 million received hospice care. Most hospice patients were female (54.7 percent), Caucasian (80.9 percent), and 65 years of age or older (84 percent). Consistent with the major causes of death in America, the majority of hospice patients had cancer (36.5 percent), dementia (15.2 percent), heart disease (13.4 percent), and lung disease (9.9 percent) (Hoyert, 2012; Kochanek, Murphy, Xu, & Arias, 2014; U.S. Centers for Disease Control and Prevention, 2015). Symptoms of disease may be acute, with death imminent by the time patients are admitted for hospice care. The NHPCO (2014, 2015a) reported that the median length of service a patient received hospice care was 17.4 days in 2014. This means that half of all hospice patients received hospice care for slightly more than 2 weeks. Approximately 35.5 percent of patients died or were discharged within 7 days after admission (see figure I.1). In 2012 an average 16.8 percent of hospice patients with Medicare died within 3 days of enrollment (Bynum, Meara, Chang, & Rhoads, 2016).

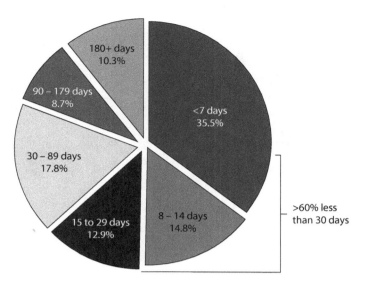

FIGURE I.1   Median length of hospice service, 2014.
Source: NHPCO (2015b).

This short length of service necessitates timely, quality hospice care so patients and their families can gain the benefits of care for as long as possible (Prince-Paul, 2008). The purpose of hospice care is to provide relief from symptoms rather than continual treatment that aims to cure a terminal illness. The Medicare hospice benefit, first established under federal law in 1982, is often the primary source of payment (NHPCO, 2015a, 2015b). Medicare-certified hospice programs are required to have an interdisciplinary team to coordinate and deliver hospice care. Hospice care is usually provided in a patient's private residence or a nursing home where a family member or designee serves as the primary caregiver. Hospice-care providers are available to see patients 24 hours a day, 7 days a week. Interdisciplinary teams consist of a physician/medical director, a registered nurse, a social worker, and a spiritual caregiver. Additional key members include home health aides, volunteers, bereavement counselors, and other therapists as needed (see figure I.2). Hospice-care providers are responsible for pain and symptom management, support for psychosocial and spiritual issues, patient access to medical supplies and equipment, family guidance in providing patient care, speech and physical therapy, coordination of inpatient

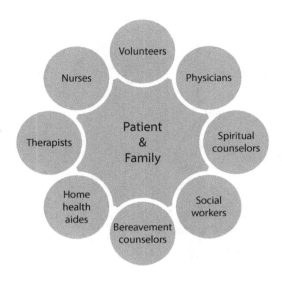

FIGURE I.2   Interdisciplinary team members.
Source: NHPCO (2015b).

admission to support symptom control, and bereavement counseling after a patient's death.

As members of interdisciplinary teams, hospice social workers share in the responsibility of ensuring patient access to biopsychosocial-spiritual care that supports the best possible quality of life and a "good death." Hospice social workers provide the majority of psychosocial services available through hospice care (Connor, 2007–2008), addressing not only a patient's psychosocial needs but also the needs of family and friends, even after a patient's death. In the process, hospice social workers provide compassionate, skilled care that builds upon patient and caregiver strengths (James, 2012; Lawson, 2007; Meier & Beresford, 2008; Puchalski, Lunsford, Harris, & Miller, 2006; Stirling, 2007). Interventions generally include patient education, crisis intervention, and supportive counseling. Social workers further enable patient and caregiver use of medical, financial, legal, and community resources involved in patient care before and after death. This requires social workers to serve as patient advocates and mediators (James, 2012). This includes ongoing assessment of how individual, family, group, organization, and community functioning influence patient well-being (Blacker & Deveau, 2010; Lawson, 2007; Meier & Beresford, 2008;

Monroe & DeLoach, 2004; Reese, 2011). Social workers are ethically responsible for ensuring all systems operate in a manner that protects, supports, and respects the rights of those who are dying (National Association of Social Workers [NASW], 2004, 2008, 2015; Payne, 2009). Some of these concerns may involve spirituality.

Hospice social workers need to be spiritually sensitive to recognize when patients need spiritual support. This is particularly important when patients highly value spirituality or religion. For example, individuals with low income or less education, those not married or living in the South, and women, racial and ethnic minorities, and older people tend to have a stronger religious affiliation (Briggs & Rayle, 2005b; Callahan, 2015; Canda & Furman, 1999, 2010; Gilligan & Furness, 2006; Hodge, 2005a, 2011; Hodge, Baughman, & Cummings, 2006; Modesto, Weaver, & Flannelly, 2006; Nelson-Becker & Canda, 2008). It is also important to recognize that spiritual needs may change as patients go through the dying process. Dying can evoke old and new spiritual challenges that require timely, quality spiritual care. Spiritual needs may require a referral to a certified hospice chaplain, but patients may not desire such a referral or the hospice might provide only limited access. A hospice social worker with the capacity to engage in spiritual care may be preferable to letting a patient's spiritual needs go unmet. Hospice social workers already address psychosocial issues that can lead to a patient's expression of spiritual concerns. In fact, according to a study conducted by Reese and Brown (1997), most issues that hospice social workers discuss with patients are spiritual in nature. Reese (2001) found that when hospice social workers address spirituality with patients, these patients actually have better outcomes. Therefore, it seems hospice social workers are already in a position to provide some form of spiritual care and may need to with certain patients. It is also reasonable to assume that by being spiritually sensitive, hospice social workers may have a more positive impact on their patients (Reese, 2013).

Spiritually sensitive hospice social work is an intervention that requires social workers to understand what spirituality means to patients and how to respond to a patient's experience of spirituality. However, what is considered an appropriate response is relative to professional boundaries, including the social worker's level of competence in addressing spiritual concerns and, most important, how spiritually supported a patient feels upon social work intervention. Hospice social workers need to be able to determine whether a patient has spiritual needs, spiritual suffering, and spiritual resources. They also need the capacity to respond in a manner that connotes spiritual competence and is, thus, experienced by the patient as being spiritually sensitive. This can occur on a generalist level by engaging patients in a therapeutic relationship that enhances a patient's experience of meaning and potential for spiritual well-being. This may further involve advanced generalist or clinical skills to help patients identify and draw from spiritual resources to address more specific spiritual needs. Collaboration with other professionals, such as a certified hospice chaplain, may be necessary to spiritually support patients (Walter, 2002). A certified hospice chaplain can address issues that are beyond a social worker's level of expertise, particularly when a patient seeks spiritual direction or has religious concerns (Hodge, 2001). Therefore, social workers can be a spiritual resource by cultivating a spiritually sensitive therapeutic relationship that may include a referral for spiritual care. Delivery of spiritually sensitive hospice social work, however, requires ongoing awareness of the spiritual dimensions of care and a willingness to ensure that hospice social workers have the spiritual competence to facilitate a patient's access to the spiritual support he or she prefers.

Although most social workers believe in the importance of addressing spirituality, research suggests that social workers feel "ambivalent about exploring spiritual and existential concerns with patients and their families" (Altilio, Gardia, & Otis-Green, 2007, p. 78; Furman, Benson, Canda, & Grimwood, 2004; Gilligan & Furness, 2006; Hodge, 2005a, 2011; Hodge & Bushfield, 2006; Nelson-Becker & Canda, 2008; Puchalski et al., 2006; Reese, 2001; Rice & McAuliffe, 2009; Sanger, 2010; Sheridan, 2009; Svare, Jay, Bruce, & Owens-Kane, 2003; Wasner, Longaker, Fegg, & Borasio, 2005). This discomfort can stem from a lack of preparation, knowledge, and time (Edwards et al., 2010; Grant, 2007; Puchalski et al., 2006; Sessanna, Finnell, Underhill, Chang, & Peng, 2011). More specifically, Puchalski et al. (2006) proposed that "many social workers are not comfortable with spiritual issues due to fears, lack of knowledge, negative associations concerning religion and spirituality, and strong feelings about separation of church and state" (p. 408). Some of this discomfort may stem from the profession's early move away from reliance on volunteers to provide moral uplift through religious charities to trained professionals who deliver evidence-based interventions through public-service organizations (Nelson-Becker & Canda, 2008; Stirling, 2007). Concerns in social work literature evolve around a desire to reduce patient risk for religious discrimination or coercion through proselytizing (Crisp, 2011). For whatever reason, being unable to address spirituality with patients when it is necessary can reduce the quality of care and increase the risk for ethical violation, if not burnout in hospice social workers (Canning, Rosenberg, & Yates, 2007; Hodge, 2011; Puchalski et al., 2006).

There has been an upward trend in social work courses that address spirituality (Hodge & McGrew, 2005; Modesto et al., 2006). Social work education has expanded insight into teaching students about spiritual diversity as a dimension of culture (Bethel, 2004; Collins, Furman, Hackman, Bender, & Bruce, 2007; Hodge & Horvath, 2011; Reese, 2013). Likewise, social work scholars have explored topics such as spiritual sensitivity, spiritual assessment, and spiritual competence (Canda & Furman, 1999, 2010; Gilligan & Furness, 2006; Hodge, 2001, 2003, 2005b; Hodge et al., 2006; Nelson-Becker & Canda, 2008; Reese, 2013; Reese, Chan, Chan, & Wiersgalla, 2010; Takahashi & Ide, 2003). Despite significant advances, more work is needed to clarify how to apply these concepts in the hospice setting. Reese (2013) stated that there are few evaluation studies that are specific to social work and spirituality and there is a need for "the development and evaluation of specific models of practice for hospice social work" (p. 49). There is also a need to build on extensive research from other disciplines. Palliative-health and nursing research has largely focused on addressing spiritual needs, spiritual pain, and spiritual care in the hospice setting (Puchalski, 2001, 2006, 2008a, 2008b, 2008c; Puchalski et al., 2006, 2009). Although some disagreement remains over how these concepts are defined, this particular body of research reflects the dominant spiritual nomenclature related to spiritual care in hospice settings (Garces-Foley, 2006; Henery, 2003a, 2003b; Pike, 2011). This book focuses on integrating research across disciplines to inform the delivery of spiritually sensitive hospice social work. This book, therefore, focuses on spirituality and hospice social work to support current and future champions of spiritual care.

CHAMPION OF SPIRITUAL CARE

Chapter 1 reflects on the importance of being a champion of spiritual care. Social workers are among those professionals charged with the responsibility of addressing the biopsychosocial-spiritual needs of hospice patients (Lawson, 2007; Parker-Oliver & Peck, 2006; Parker-Oliver, Bronstein, &

Kurzejeski, 2005;). Starting with Cicely Saunders, a trained social worker, nurse, and doctor, multiple disciplines have been considered essential for the delivery of quality hospice care. The fields of medicine and nursing have expanded research on spirituality with new work in the field of social work to build spiritual competence (Barber, 2012). Spiritual competence is grounded on the ability of hospice social workers to be spiritually sensitive and prepared to facilitate patient access to timely spiritual care by referral, if not directly. Such preparedness is necessary in case a patient expresses an urgent need for spiritual care or refuses a referral to a formal spiritual-care provider or both. The work of Hodge (2011) and associates (Hodge & Bushfield, 2006; Hodge et al., 2006) suggests that building spiritual competence is a continuous process that involves an awareness of the individual's own worldview and assumptions, empathic understanding of a patient's worldview, and interventions that are sensitive to a patient's worldview. Hospice social workers can build spiritual competence as practitioner-learners on interdisciplinary teams. This practice enhances the ability of hospice social workers to communicate in a spiritually sensitive manner with patients and create spiritually sensitive conditions in the treatment environment so other interdisciplinary team members may develop spiritual competence (Canda & Furman, 1999, 2010). In the process of being champions of spiritual care, hospice social workers can enhance the overall quality of hospice care and, most importantly, the quality of life for patients and their families facing terminal illness.

SPIRITUAL DIVERSITY

Chapter 2 examines a variety of perspectives about what defines spirituality. Some of these perspectives may inform patients' and hospice social workers' worldviews, as spirituality is considered a social construct. It is the tradition of social work to value the dignity and worth of each person. This includes maintaining respect for patients with different religious and spiritual beliefs (Krieglstein, 2006). Part of this includes being aware of what a patient wants and needs for spiritual support, because the dying process can lead to questions about the meaning of life and what follows after death (McSherry, Cash, & Ross, 2004; Puchalski et al., 2006). Addressing spiritual issues, like psychosocial issues, is not a routinized process; needs and resources evolve over time. For example, what informs spiritual needs starts with how one defines spirituality. The dominant view that each person is on a unique spiritual journey reflects a Judeo-Christian, Western understanding of spirituality (Sessanna et al., 2011; Weatherby, 2002). Hence, the conceptualization of any experience is relative to an individual's worldview, making the definition of spirituality culture-dependent (Weatherby, 2002). Social workers need to create the space for patients to shape their own spiritual narrative. In the context of this spiritual discourse, social workers can work toward understanding a patient's worldview. This is particularly important when a patient's worldview differs from the dominant culture (Chatters & Taylor, 2003; Gay, Lynxwiler, & Peek, 2001; Wright, 2002). Even if a social worker identifies with a patient's particular religious group or is from a similar sociocultural background, there may be fundamental differences in how the patient defines spirituality and the importance of religious beliefs that are "pivotal for well being" (Chatters & Taylor, 2003, p. 145). Hence, in the process of understanding a patient's worldview, it helps to be able to reference various ways spirituality has been conceptualized. It is this process of seeking spiritual understanding that allows for spiritual sensitivity to emerge.

SPIRITUAL NEEDS

Chapter 3 explores potential spiritual needs associated with dying. Research will provide the foundation for this discussion, particularly in how individual factors seem to shape a patient's spiritual needs. Patients can experience spiritual needs regardless of whether a disease is chronic or becomes terminal. As described by Doka (2011), in the beginning, patients have to cope with the fear of being diagnosed with a life-threatening disease. However expected, diagnosis may come as a shock and evoke fear as the disease threatens one's very existence. Physical vulnerability exposes the fragility of life. This can lead to questions such as "Why me?" and "Why now?" as a person struggles to understand. Life becomes divided into before and after the diagnosis. During the chronic phase, a patient may have to find new ways to cope with symptoms of the disease and side effects of treatment. One may resume normal activities, social roles, and responsibilities, although social supports may not be as available as they were when first diagnosed. Spiritual questions may return, such as, "Is this treatment worth the suffering?" and "What does my future hold?" Moral or ethical decisions will need to be made about life-sustaining measures with support potentially from spiritual leaders. Some patients may view suffering as a punishment for sins, and others may consider suffering an opportunity for transcendence. The chronic phase can lead to recovery, perhaps considered a blessing that requires one to live a better life. Patients may reject their spiritual community because they feel abandoned during illness. When illness progresses into the terminal phase, treatment changes from efforts to cure the disease to measures to reduce the symptoms of disease. At this time, patients are said to struggle the most with three spiritual needs. The first need is to assess life as having meaning and purpose, which may entail seeking forgiveness or reconciliation. The second need is to die in a preferred manner, described as "a good death" free from suffering. The third need is to experience hope that one's life will continue through being remembered by others or having descendants who will carry on the family name or community work that stands in memorial. Despite the guise of a predictable trajectory, spiritual needs are not always predictable.

SPIRITUAL SUFFERING

Chapter 4 discusses how patients may be at risk for unmet spiritual needs and spiritual suffering. This includes discussion about facilitating patient access to spiritual resources to build or sustain spiritual resilience. However the dying process unfolds, patients facing life-limiting illness have the potential to experience spiritual needs that can lead to spiritual suffering (Belcher & Griffiths, 2005; Harrington, 2004; Hodge & Horvath, 2011; Miller, Chibnall, Videen, & Duckro, 2005; Nelson-Becker & Canda, 2008; Puchalski, 2001). Therefore it is particularly important for hospice social workers to better understand how patients view spirituality, including spiritual resources that promote spiritual resilience. Millison (1988) defines spiritual needs as a desire "to integrate goals, values, and experiences in search of meaning and sense of purpose" (pp. 37–38). The process of making these connections is believed to enable patients to better understand how they fit in the world and the implications of death. The ability to come to terms with the reality of terminal illness reflects a form of spiritual coping. When patients have difficulty integrating life experiences in a manner that supports life satisfaction, this unmet spiritual need for meaning can increase the risk of spiritual suffering. Hence, based on this perspective, spiritual suffering is existential in nature and arises from the failure to find meaning in life in the face of pending death. This experience of spiritual suffering may lead to detachment from others, confusion, or hopelessness. For example, spiritual suffering may be expressed through a patient's struggle with questions such as "Why is this happening to me?," "What is the meaning of my life?," and "Do others value me and see me as a person of worth?" (Bratton, 2005; Knight & von Gunten, 2004b; McCormick, 2007; Puchalski, 2008c; Wintz & Cooper, 2003). Therefore, the struggle to cope can lead to spiritual suffering, also known as a spiritual crisis or spiritual emergency (Sperry & Miller, 2010). A failure to support patients can leave them vulnerable to spiritual suffering, which can compromise overall well-being (Balboni et al., 2007; Hermann, 2007; Koenig, 2007) and lead to increased use of services that fail to address the spiritual cause of distress (Grant et al., 2004).

RELATIONAL SPIRITUALITY

Chapter 5 focuses on how relational spirituality may emerge through a therapeutic relationship. In this way, hospice social workers can help patients cultivate or sustain spiritual resilience. Therapeutic relationships can influence client outcomes, and evidence suggests that particular aspects of the relational process are key (Skovholt, 2005). Qualities and skills such as empathy and generosity can have a significant influence over therapeutic outcomes regardless of treatment approach (Feller & Cottone, 2003). Preliminary research on relational depth demonstrates that social worker and patient may both be changed by a therapeutic encounter (Cooper, 2005; Knox, 2008). This necessitates a balance between detachment and closeness through skillful use of professional boundaries. Relationships also have spiritual dimensions that are often not named (McGrath & Newell, 2004). Rather than relying on words, spirituality may be best understood experientially through relationships that make life more meaningful. It is natural for patients to have "the human need to transcend, to go beyond the suffering and to find meaning in that experience" (Kellehear, 2000, p. 153). Relationships with self and others may facilitate this need to move beyond suffering to spiritual resilience and shared healing. Cultivating a spiritual awareness of one's connection with the environment may be just as important. Therefore, all types of relationships have the potential to evoke spiritual experiences, suggesting a spirituality rooted in relationships. This type of spirituality may likewise be experienced in the social work relationship (Sandage & Shults, 2007). Based on interviews with 50 social service providers and advocates, Faver (2004) found that one's engagement in caregiving facilitated a "joy and vitality" that went beyond satisfaction with outcomes (p. 243). It was suggested that relational spirituality involved the process of relating to others through care provision and not only strengthened relationships but also enhanced one's spiritual capacity to sustain care. Callahan (2015) further described relational spirituality as the experience of enhanced life meaning through a morally fulfilling relationship with the self, someone/something else, or a higher power, which may be experienced by both patient and social worker through a spiritually sensitive therapeutic relationship.

SPIRITUAL CARE

Chapter 6 defines spiritual care and how spiritually sensitive hospice social work may further serve as a resource for spiritual care. Spiritual care has traditionally fallen under the auspices of chaplains. Social workers are among the hospice professionals who have joined chaplains in the provision of spiritual care. Spiritual care involves delivering compassionate care that is sensitive to what clients want and need spiritually (Chochinov & Cann, 2005; Daaleman, Usher, Williams, Rawlings, & Hanson, 2008; MacConville, 2006; Peteet & Balboni, 2013; Puchalski, 2001; Stephenson, Draucker, & Martsolf, 2003; Swinton & Pattison, 2010; Wright, 2002). Spiritual care is not intended to provide answers to unanswerable questions but to open spiritual dialogues that meet the spiritual needs of patients. Clients have unique spiritual needs as well as spiritual resources that can promote spiritual resilience. For example, with hospice clients, spiritual care "involves forging meaningful connections, respecting the clients' choices for managing their dying, and eliciting stories about life and death" (Stephenson et al., 2003, p. 51). This may require the building of spiritual competence to facilitate an "activity" or "series of tasks" that support a client's "quest" for spiritual well-being. Given the centrality of relationship in social work practice, social workers may cultivate a spiritually sensitive relationship that can serve as a form of spiritual care. This necessitates a move away from the religious care that has been traditionally delivered by chaplains to other ways of facilitating spiritual care that fall under the auspices of hospice social work. Traditional social work skills may be used in the delivery of spiritual care, but this also demands a heightened level of spiritual sensitivity, willingness to build spiritual competence, and interdisciplinary collaboration to ensure a patient's spiritual needs are met. Holloway, Adamson, McSherry, and Swinton (2011) broadly categorized 12 different spiritual care models as conceptual, competency, whole-person synergy, interdisciplinary, or organizational, with some degree of overlap between. These models demonstrate how factors such as hospice social worker and patient characteristics may influence the spiritual care process and provide a foundation for the application of Callahan's (2013) relational model for spiritually sensitive hospice social work.

SPIRITUAL SENSITIVITY

Chapter 7 examines what defines spiritual sensitivity and how hospice social work may employ the relational model for spiritually sensitive hospice social work. Canda and Furman (1999) described spiritual sensitivity as "a way of being and relating throughout the entire helping process" that provides a foundation for good social work practice but requires intentional efforts to sustain "a spiritual vision of human capacity and possibility" (pp. 186, 283). Canda (1999) suggested spiritual sensitivity inspires unconditional love, compassion, and a genuine desire to help patients. Social workers who seek to treat patients as "full and complete persons, with inherent worthiness of respect . . . rather than diagnostic categories or bundles of problems or dysfunctions" are spiritually sensitive (p. 9). Building on this work, Callahan (2013, 2015) proposed that hospice social workers have the ability to cultivate a therapeutic relationship that is experienced as life enhancing for a patient. Spiritually sensitive hospice social work is an intervention model that honors the dignity and worth of the patient. This requires the provision of care that is congruent with a patient's spiritual or religious worldview based on, for example, a patient's definition of spirituality, spiritual needs, spiritual suffering, and spiritual resources. Hospice social workers can draw from generalist, advanced generalist, or clinical skills to serve as a spiritual resource. Generalist skills are inherent in any spiritually sensitive relationship given the relational qualities that are needed to convey compassion and inspire enhanced life meaning; however, the building of spiritual competence may be needed for the direct delivery of spiritual care, if not a referral to a professional with more expertise.

Hence, spiritually sensitive hospice social work may serve as a form of spiritual care if patients feel spiritually supported through the therapeutic relationship, even if awareness of such is just for a moment.

SPIRITUAL COMPETENCE

Chapter 8 stresses the importance of spiritual competence as a means of evaluating spiritually sensitive hospice social work and ends with a renewed charge for hospice social workers to be champions of quality spiritual care. In 2011, the Council on Social Work Education (2015a) created the Religion and Spirituality Work Group to help social workers learn more about diverse expressions of spirituality. Spiritual competence is a more specific form of cultural competence (Hodge et al., 2006; Hodge & Bushfield, 2006). Like cultural competence, spiritual competence requires social workers to understand how spirituality may shape human behavior and be a source of strength, how spiritual diversity manifests in society and can enhance risk for discrimination, and how to build relationships that are spiritually sensitive (NASW, 2008, 2015). Spiritual competence has been described as ranging on a continuum. Spiritual competence is on one end, and a lack of spiritual competence, which may reflect spiritual insensitivity and in some cases spiritually destructive practices, is on the other end of the continuum (Hodge et al., 2006). For example, hospice social workers need spiritual competence if a patient requests prayer. Spiritual competence decreases the risk of praying with a patient without regard for the patient's worldview. Hence, spiritual sensitivity requires the capacity to recognize one's level of spiritual competence. There are a number of social work and related models that detail competencies required for spiritual competence. The work of Hodge (2011) and associates (Hodge & Bushfield, 2006; Hodge et al., 2006) can be used to help clarify what spiritual competence means for hospice social workers. This work approaches the building of spiritual competence as a continuous process that involves an awareness of the individual's own worldview and assumptions, empathic understanding of a patient's worldview, and interventions that are sensitive to a patient's worldview. Since relationships are essential in facilitating spiritual support, these relationships are likely to include interdisciplinary teamwork. Therefore, the work of Puchalski and colleagues (2009) further clarifies how hospice social workers may be a spiritual resource for and with interdisciplinary team members.

PART | **1**

Understanding Key Components

1

Champion of Spiritual Care

HOSPICE SOCIAL WORKERS HAVE BEEN members of interdisciplinary teams with the responsibility of providing holistic care since the beginning of the hospice movement. Each team member has an area of expertise, with hospice social workers being primarily responsible for the delivery of psychosocial care (Connor, 2007–2008). Although certified hospice chaplains are primarily responsible for the delivery of spiritual care, as interdisciplinary team members, hospice social workers must be prepared to ensure patients have access to the spiritual care they prefer. A hospice social worker can be a spiritual resource by cultivating a spiritually sensitive therapeutic relationship that may lead to a referral for or delivery of spiritual care. It can be difficult to address a patient's spiritual needs, particularly when those needs are ambiguous in nature and are likely to change as part of the dying process. Nevertheless, the need for a timely response requires hospice social workers who are spiritually sensitive to respond independently and in coordination with interdisciplinary team members for patient access to quality spiritual care. This chapter will highlight the essential role of hospice social workers as champions of spiritual care.

LIFE QUALITY UNTIL DEATH

Palliative care is coordinated interdisciplinary care for patients with a serious chronic illness; it strives to promote the best quality of life for patients and their families (Payne, 2009; Puchalski et al., 2009). Palliative care adds an "extra layer of support" for symptom management as care providers work in conjunction with a patient's regular physician (Center to Advance Palliative Care, 2012, p. 2). When an illness is no longer curable and is certified by a physician as being likely to lead to death within six months, a patient may elect hospice care, which is a form of palliative care (Almgren, n.d.; Centers for Medicare & Medicaid Services [CMS], n.d.; Monroe & DeLoach, 2004). This approach continues to provide biopsychosocial-spiritual resources but focuses on cultivating an environment that honors a patient's need for dignity, self-determination, and comfort throughout the dying process (Clark et al., 2007; Frank, 2009; Monroe & DeLoach, 2004; Oliver, Washington, Wittenberg-Lyles, & Demiris, 2009). In providing hospice care, there are four primary objectives that include (1) promoting comfort essential for maintaining life quality; (2) allowing for self-determination congruent with patient culture, values, and lifestyle; (3) creating opportunities for growth in keeping with the developmental challenges associated with the end of life; and (4) meeting the multidimensional needs of patients and caregiver(s) (Parker-Oliver & Peck, 2006). As such, an interdisciplinary team is necessary to coordinate a multiskilled effort to address patient biopsychosocial-spiritual needs (Muehlbauer, 2013). This not only involves the work of multiple professionals but also informal caregivers over the course of illness (Bliss & While, 2007; Monroe & DeLoach, 2004; Payne, 2009).

INTERDISCIPLINARY TEAMS

Joint efforts between multiple professionals and informal caregivers have long been a part of the therapeutic quality of hospice care (Monroe & DeLoach, 2004; Parker-Oliver & Peck, 2006). The hospice movement began in 1967 with the opening of Saint Christopher's Hospice in England by Cicely Saunders. Efforts to reform health care for the terminally ill in the United States began in 1973 under the direction of Florence Wald (Lawson, 2007). The hospice movement was founded on the belief that patients needed the services of different professionals during the dying process (Parker-Oliver, Bronstein, & Kurzejeski, 2005; Parker-Oliver & Peck, 2006). Saunders herself was trained as a social worker, nurse, and doctor. This interdisciplinary approach was further established when the U.S. Congress first authorized a hospice benefit under Medicare in 1982 and private health insurance companies and the Veterans Administration began to pay for hospice care (Almgren, n.d.; National Hospice and Palliative Care Organization [NHPCO], 2015a; Oliver et al., 2009). The Joint Commission began accrediting hospice providers, which further established Medicare-certified hospices to provide services through an interdisciplinary team that includes a registered nurse, social worker, and spiritual caregiver under the supervision of a physician (CMS, n.d.; Condition of Participation: Core Services, 2010; Joint Commission, 2016; Lawson, 2007). Membership may be extended to ancillary staff, such as home health aides and informal caregivers (Monroe & DeLoach, 2004; Muehlbauer, 2013; Oliver et al., 2009; Parker-Oliver et al., 2005). To help ensure hospice care remains responsive to patient needs, the Joint Commission requires a patient's care plan be reviewed and updated during interdisciplinary team meetings at least every 15 days (Oliver et al., 2009). Hence, hospice care requires collaboration for intervention (Monroe & DeLoach, 2004).

Team collaboration involves a synergistic interaction between professionals with a range of perspectives and skills (Blacker & Deveau, 2010; Parker-Oliver et al., 2005). As described by Blacker and Deveau (2010), interdisciplinary team members are responsible for patient-centered care that involves (1) assessing patient condition, (2) helping patients understand the trajectory of illness, (3) assisting patients in making decisions, (4) connecting patients to resources, and (5) helping caregiver(s) manage the consequences of illness. In the process, according to Payne (2006), an interdisciplinary team is an interpersonal space in which a "community of practice" emerges (p. 138). Interdisciplinary teams generally streamline service provision by connecting patients with the most appropriate professionals to ensure patient needs are met (Blacker & Deveau, 2010; Lawson, 2007). This requires thoughtful cultivation of mutual respect among interdisciplinary team members that starts with an understanding of each member's professional roles and competencies (Blacker & Deveau, 2010; Lawson, 2007; Wittenberg-Lyles, Parker-Oliver, Demiris, Baldwin, & Regehr, 2008; Payne, 2006). This process has the potential to shape formal and informal roles, give meaning to work relationships, forge a sense of belonging, and build a commitment to care that prevents burnout (Blacker & Deveau, 2010). This presupposes work conditions that allow for a collaborative process to emerge. Team members need the flexibility to stretch professional boundaries to support patient care (Blacker & Deveau, 2010; Payne, 2006). It is through this process of team collaboration that members share in responsibility for assessment, planning, intervention, and outcomes, all of which inform the quality of care (Clark et al., 2007; James, 2012; Lamers, 2007; Lawson, 2007; Parker-Oliver et al., 2005).

More research is needed to measure the effect of interdisciplinary teamwork; however, it is generally believed that good team collaboration enhances the quality of hospice care (Auty, 2005; Goldsmith, Wittenberg-Lyles, Rodriguez, & Sanchez-Reilly, 2010; Parker-Oliver et al., 2005; Payne, 2006; Reese, 2011b; Wittenberg-Lyles et al., 2008). For example, in a national survey based on a random sample of 66 hospices, Reese and Raymer (2004) found that team collaboration correlated with fewer than average hospitalizations and lower overall hospice costs. Goldsmith et al. (2010) found that team collaboration enhanced symptom control and patient satisfaction. Conversely, poor collaboration between interdisciplinary team members can compromise service provision. Different disciplines may have stereotyped views of one another (Auty, 2005). Even when professional roles are distinguished, role ambiguity and conflict can still occur (Blacker & Deveau, 2010; Wittenberg-Lyles et al., 2008). This is particularly true for social workers and spiritual caregivers, whose roles may not be as clear (James, 2012). Turf issues may also arise when team members cover for one another (Lawson, 2007). For example, Medicare does not require hospice organizations to employ hospice chaplains on interdisciplinary teams, so other spiritual caregivers as well as interdisciplinary team members may share in this work (Condition of Participation: Core Services, 2010). Wittenberg-Lyles et al. (2008) found that one-third (35 percent) of chaplains reported having experienced role conflict with either social workers (19 percent) or nurses (14 percent). Hence, additional efforts may be required to coordinate responsibilities for spiritual-care provision (Blacker & Deveau, 2010; James, 2012). Despite these challenges, team members can learn from one another and gain a broader understanding of patient needs as they work together (Blacker & Deveau, 2010; Clark et al., 2007; Goldsmith et al., 2010; Lamers, 2007; Parker-Oliver et al., 2005). Team members can further provide services that complement one another's work and multiply the resources available to patients.

SOCIAL WORKERS AS TEAM MEMBERS

Professional roles, group norms, and organizational factors can influence the collaborative process (Goldsmith et al., 2010; Payne, 2006; Wittenberg-Lyles et al., 2008). Social workers have a range of competencies that enable them to be essential interdisciplinary team members across treatment settings. In hospice care, social workers have been team members since the beginning of the hospice movement and later, as per Medicare rules (CMS, n.d.; Condition of Participation: Core Services, 2010; Holloway, Adamson, McSherry, & Swinton, 2011; Parker-Oliver et al., 2005; Lawson, 2007). Hospice social workers have been described as being "at the heart of palliative care" (Stirling, 2007, p. 24), for they provide compassionate, skilled care that builds on patient and caregiver strengths to promote psychosocial-spiritual well-being (Connor, 2007–2008; James, 2012; Lawson, 2007; Meier & Beresford, 2008; Puchalski, Lunsford, Harris, & Miller, 2006). Intervention starts with an assessment of patient needs and resources that inform care planning, treatment, and referral. Social workers seek information about, for example, psychological challenges anticipated with grief and the influence of family dynamics and other social systems that broadly include culture. Death and dying can have implications for families and communities that may require social workers to build on family resilience and community capacity. Social work intervention generally includes patient education, crisis intervention, and supportive counseling. Social workers further enable caregiver use of medical, financial, legal, and community resources to support patient care and bereavement after death. This includes social work intervention as patient advocacy and mediation and coordination with team members for timely access to care (James, 2012; Monroe & DeLoach, 2004).

Social workers are responsible for ensuring treatment conditions support life quality (Gert, Culver, & Clouser, 2006; National Association of Social Workers [NASW], 2004, 2008; Payne, 2009). This involves ongoing assessment of how social systems, including interdisciplinary teams, influence patient well-being (Blacker & Deveau, 2010; Lawson, 2007; Meier & Beresford, 2008; Monroe & DeLoach, 2004; Reese, 2011b). On interdisciplinary teams, hospice social workers are needed to help team members see how multiple dimensions inform this process. For example, social workers may address the nonphysical aspects of pain as described by Terry Altilio, a leader in hospice social work, in Meier and Beresford (2008):

> "When you look at pain from a multidimensional perspective—not to minimize the importance of physical aspects of pain management—there is meaning to the symptoms of illness for the patient and family. There are emotional consequences of uncontrolled pain and spiritual issues: Does this patient feel that pain is redemptive—or a punishment from God? Some patients feel that pain means they are dying. If we don't ask patients about what the illness and the symptoms mean to them, we never hear their worst fears." Pain and suffering also cause enormous distress for family members. There can be fear and anticipation of witnessing suffering in a loved one, and concerns about the social–economic aspects of pain, such as the huge costs of many analgesics. "People tend to talk to social workers in a different way, because we don't 'do things' procedurally, write orders or give medications," Altilio says. Social workers experienced in pain management also bring skills such as relaxation therapy, guided imagery or cognitive restructuring to help patients feel more in control of their symptom experiences. "Pain management is a shared responsibility with our colleagues," Altilio says. "I have profound respect for doctors' and nurses' training and expertise. But as social workers, we bring a different view of the world. We're trained to see the situation in a way that integrates the physical with the psychosocial–spiritual.
>
> (p. 12)

Therefore, a multidimensional, systems perspective makes social workers uniquely qualified to serve on interdisciplinary teams (Parker-Oliver et al., 2005; Payne, 2009). In addition to recognizing a patient's needs on the micro level, social workers see the consequences of the dying process on the mezzo and macro levels through patient caregivers and friends. This involves facilitating access to psychosocial services that may extend to spiritual care. Part of this responsibility is to support good team functioning by employing coordination and mediation skills and education and advocacy skills to ensure patient access to quality hospice care (Meier & Beresford, 2008; Stirling, 2007).

Not only are social workers essential members of interdisciplinary care teams, social work services are linked to positive treatment outcomes and reduced costs (Reese, 2011b, 2013). Reese and Raymer (2004) found that having qualified social workers on interdisciplinary teams allowed for better team functioning. Social workers were able to address more issues with the teams, particularly when the social workers were only responsible for providing social work services. This was also significantly correlated with a reduced need for patient visits by other team members. The authors suggested that social workers facilitated early identification of patient risk for psychosocial crisis, intervention to meet psychosocial needs, and better communication with hospice staff. Most importantly, social workers were positively related to patient satisfaction. The extent of social work involvement, however, is likely to be related to professional expertise. Reese (2011b) conducted a national survey of hospice directors ($n = 43$) to see whether there were any changes in social work utilization compared with the results of an earlier study by Kulys and Davis (1986, 1987). Social workers were still perceived to be the most qualified to provide financial counseling (98 percent) and make referrals (83 percent); however, new areas of expertise emerged. Social workers were considered qualified to conduct an intake interview (75 percent), facilitate social support (66 percent), promote cultural competence (54 percent), and facilitate community outreach (50 percent). Social workers were also considered to be the most qualified to perform counseling, particularly when patients wanted to hasten death (67 percent) or were in denial of impending death (54 percent).

Of greatest concern, Reese found that social workers were considered qualified to perform only half of the interventions they were trained to perform (12 out of 24). Seventy-nine percent of hospice directors viewed psychosocial assessment to be within a social worker's role, but only 21 percent viewed social workers as being the most qualified to perform this role. Social workers were not considered qualified to address the spiritual experiences of patients (0 percent) and minimally qualified to discuss the meaning of life (19 percent). However, in Reese and Raymer (2004), family functioning was predicted by the number of spiritual issues addressed by social workers and whether the social workers had arranged spiritual support. Although social workers were considered qualified to promote cultural competence (54 percent), they were considered minimally qualified to ensure culturally competent end-of-life decisions (14 percent). It was not clear why social workers were considered minimally qualified to ensure culturally competent end-of-life decisions, but it seems inconsistent and contrary to instilling confidence in culturally competent hospice social work. In fact, the spiritual caregiver was considered qualified for ensuring culturally competent end-of-life decisions, which suggests some relationship between cultural and spiritual competence (52 percent). Culturally competent hospice social work requires sensitivity to all dimensions of the human experience, including the spiritual dimension. In addition to being required for ethical social work practice (NASW, 2004, 2008, 2015; Council on Social Work Education [CSWE], 2008, 2015a, 2015b, 2015c), culturally competent services are required by Medicare to offset risk for treatment disparities throughout the provision of hospice care (CMS, 2012; Hospice Foundation of America [HFA], 2011; NHPCO, n.d., b). Any disconnection between professional training and perceived competence would likely have implications for team performance and patient access to quality hospice care.

PROFESSIONAL FOUNDATION

Since the 1980s the profession of social work has taken important steps to improve social work expertise in end-of-life care (Reese, 2011b). The Project on Death in America (PDIA) was one initiative that sponsored the advancement of social work research and practice in this area. The PDIA was a program managed by the Open Society Institute, now called Open Society Foundations, established by George Soros (OSF, 2015). The PDIA provided grants to individuals and organizations to advance end-of-life care (OSI, 2004). The PDIA, along with the Robert Wood Johnson Foundation and Duke Institute on Care at the End of Life, sponsored a Social Work Leadership Summit on End-of-Life and Palliative Care in 2002 (Altilio et al., 2007). This event provided a forum for social workers to report on the state of social work practice, research, education, and policy and to further delineate plans to advance quality end-of-life care (Altilio et al., 2007; Blacker, Christ, & Lynch, n.d.). In 2005 a second Social Work Leadership Summit sponsored by the PDIA and hosted by the NASW with support from the NHPCO was provided for participants to share accomplishments since the first summit and to clarify additional priorities and partnerships (Altilio et al., 2007).

These summits established a momentum that continues to promote quality end-of-life care. There were conference presentations, special-issue journal publications, online listservs, newsletters, curricular and teaching materials, continuing education opportunities, establishment of a new journal (called the *Journal of Social Work in End-of-Life Care*), and funding for research that more than doubled PDIA's initial investment (Blacker et al., n.d.). Another important accomplishment was the development of the *NASW Standards for Social Work Practice in Palliative and End of Life Care* in 2004. These standards have provided guidelines for the appropriate ethics/values, knowledge, assessment, intervention/treatment planning, attitude/self-awareness, empowerment/advocacy, documentation, interdisciplinary teamwork, cultural competence, continuing education, and supervision/leadership/training for social workers who engage in end-of-life care. The Social Work Hospice and Palliative Care Network (SWHPN) was also established later in 2007 to help coordinate a coalition of experts and facilitate collaboration between organizations that support social workers in providing quality palliative and hospice care. Among other things, for example, the SWHPN (2013) provides social workers a clearinghouse for resources with an annual conference that provides educational and networking opportunities.

A parallel movement was the creation in 2001 of the National Consensus Project (NCP) for Quality Palliative Care by a group of interdisciplinary experts who sought to standardize and improve the quality of hospice and palliative care nationwide. This group developed *Clinical Guidelines for Quality Palliative Care*, which included eight domains of care defined by guidelines with specific criteria to fulfill each guideline (NCP, 2013). These eight domains include structure/processes, physical, psychological and psychiatric, social, spiritual/religious/existential, cultural, care of the patient at the end of life, and ethical/legal aspects of care. As part of the second Social Work Leadership Summit on End-of-Life and Palliative Care, a committee of social workers conducted a thorough review of these NCP standards and practices to determine whether they were congruent with social work knowledge based on the work of leaders in the field. They found that the NCP guidelines provided social workers "a solid base on which to build specialized expertise in palliative and end-of-life care" (Blacker et al., n.d., p. 12). The NASW was involved in the revision of these clinical guidelines. Such efforts not only punctuated the importance of social work involvement but also the investment of professional social work organizations in supporting the delivery of quality palliative and end-of-life care. This further suggests social work leaders recognize that palliative and end-of-life care may require social workers to be sensitive to the spiritual, religious, and existential issues of patients and, thus, necessitate spiritual competence.

The NCP also worked with the National Quality Forum (NQF), a nonprofit membership organization that promotes national standards for health-care improvement, to advance evidence-based palliative care. The NCP guidelines in box 1.1 and NQF preferred practices in box 1.2 are guidelines for spiritual care across disciplines. The NQF built on the NCP *Clinical Guidelines for Quality Palliative Care* to develop a set of preferred practices with measurable outcomes (NCP, 2013; NQF, 2006). This document was later revised and a second edition published in 2009. The most recent third edition was released in 2013 (NCP, 2013). In short, as seen in box 1.2, the NQF (2006) provides four preferred practices (practices 20 to 23) that address the spiritual, religious, and existential aspects of end-of-life care. Practice 20 calls for expertise in using an instrument for the assessment of religious, spiritual, and existential concerns and the integration of such information into care planning. Practice 21 expects spiritual-care services to be made available through the hospice organization or patient clergy, which would require awareness of such resources and ability to make referrals and coordinate care to meet spiritual needs. Practice 22 is likely to be accomplished by default if the hospice organization employs a spiritual caregiver as required by Medicare, although the level of training is at the discretion of the employer, which would likely influence access to quality spiritual care. Practice 23 requires spiritual-care providers to build relationships with community clergy and provide education and counseling to meet patient spiritual needs. Hospice social workers share in the responsibility for all of these practices in coordination with interdisciplinary team members.

Social workers must be sensitive to the religious, spiritual, and existential beliefs of patients as an extension of cultural competence (Fukuyama & Sevig, 1997; Hodge et al., 2006). The *Indicators for the Achievement of the NASW Standards for Cultural Competence in Social Work Practice* (2001, 2015), also referenced in the *NASW Standards for Social Work Practice in Palliative and End of Life Care* (2004) (see box 1.3), states that a patient's "history, traditions, values" and how he or she is influenced by his or her "ethnicity, culture, values, religion- and health-related beliefs, and economic situations" must be considered by social workers in the practice of end-of-life

Guideline 5.1 The interdisciplinary team assesses and addresses spiritual,
religious, and existential dimensions of care.

Criteria

Spirituality is recognized as a fundamental aspect of compassionate, patient and
family centered care that honors the dignity of all persons.

- Spirituality is defined as "the aspect of humanity that refers to the way
individuals seek and express meaning and purpose and the way they experience
their connectedness to the moment, to self, to others, to nature, and/or to the
significant or sacred." It is the responsibility of all IDT [interdisciplinary team]
members to recognize spiritual distress and attend to the patient's and the family's spiritual needs, within their scope of practice.
- The interdisciplinary palliative care team, in all settings, includes spiritual
care professionals; ideally a board certified professional chaplain, with skill and
expertise to assess and address spiritual and existential issues frequently confronted by pediatric and adult patients with life-threatening or serious illnesses
and their families.
- Communication with the patient and family is respectful of their religious
and spiritual beliefs, rituals, and practices. Palliative care team members do not
impose their individual spiritual, religious, existential beliefs, or practices on patients, families, or colleagues.

Guideline 5.2 A spiritual assessment process, including a spiritual screening,
history questions, and a full spiritual assessment as indicated, is performed. This
assessment identifies religious or spiritual/existential background, preferences,
and related beliefs, rituals, and practices of the patient and family, as well as
symptoms, such as spiritual distress and/or pain, guilt, resentment, despair,
and hopelessness.

Criteria

- The IDT regularly explores spiritual and existential concerns and documents these spiritual themes in order to communicate them to the team. This
exploration includes, but is not limited to: life review, assessment of hopes,

BOX 1.1 *(CONTINUED)*

values, and fears, meaning, purpose, beliefs about afterlife, spiritual or religious practices, cultural norms, beliefs that influence understanding of illness, coping, guilt, forgiveness, and life completion tasks. Whenever possible, a standardized instrument is used.

- The IDT periodically reevaluates the impact of spiritual/existential interventions and documents patient and family preferences.
- The patient's spiritual resources of strength are supported and documented in the patient record.
- Spiritual/existential care needs, goals, and concerns identified by patients, family members, the palliative care team, or spiritual care professionals are addressed according to established protocols and documented in the interdisciplinary care plan, and emphasized during transitions of care, and/or in discharge plans. Support is offered for issues of life closure, as well as other spiritual issues, in a manner consistent with the patient's and the family's cultural, spiritual, and religious values.
- Referral to an appropriate community-based professional with specialized knowledge or skills in spiritual and existential issues (e.g., to a pastoral counselor or spiritual director) is made when desired by the patient and/or family. Spiritual care professionals are recognized as specialists who provide spiritual counseling.

Guideline 5.3 The palliative care service facilitates religious, spiritual, and cultural rituals or practices as desired by patient and family, especially at and after the time of death.

Criteria

- Professional and institutional use of religious/spiritual symbols and language are sensitive to cultural and religious diversity.
- The patient and family are supported in their desires to display and use their own religious/spiritual and/or cultural symbols.
- Chaplaincy and other palliative care professionals facilitate contact with spiritual/religious communities, groups or individuals, as desired by the patient and/or family. Palliative care programs create procedures to facilitate patients' access to clergy, religious, spiritual and culturally-based leaders, and/or healers in their own religious, spiritual, or cultural traditions.

BOX 1.1 *(CONTINUED)*

• Palliative professionals acknowledge their own spirituality as part of their professional role. Opportunities are provided to engage staff in self-care and self-reflection of their beliefs and values as they work with seriously ill and dying patients. Core expectations of the team include respect of spirituality and beliefs of all colleagues and the creation of a healing environment in the workplace.

• Non-chaplain palliative care providers obtain training in basic spiritual screening and spiritual care skills.

• The palliative care team ensures postdeath follow up after the patient's death (e.g. phone calls, attendance at wake or funeral, or scheduled visit) to offer support, identify any additional needs that require community referral, and help the family during bereavement.

Clinical Implications

Spiritual, religious, and existential issues are a fundamental aspect of quality of life for patients with serious or life-threatening illness and their families. All team members are accountable for attending to spiritual care in a respectful fashion. In order to provide an optimal and inclusive healing environment, each palliative care team member needs to be aware of his or her own spirituality and how it may differ from fellow team members and those of the patients and families they serve.

Source: NCP (2013).

BOX 1.2 SPIRITUAL, RELIGIOUS, AND EXISTENTIAL ASPECTS OF PALLIATIVE CARE: NATIONAL QUALITY FORUM PREFERRED PRACTICES

Domain 5. Spiritual, religious, and existential aspects of care.

Under the stressful conditions of the palliative care setting, the patient's and family's concerns about religious and spiritual matters become of paramount importance. Programs must be able to assess these needs and provide appropriate resources to meet them.

The Problem

Spirituality is an important, yet often neglected, factor in the health of hospitalized patients. Up to 77 percent of patients would like spiritual issues considered as part

BOX 1.2 (CONTINUED)

of their medical care, yet only 10 to 20 percent of physicians discuss these issues with their patients. Other studies indicate that although nurses also have frequent interactions with patients receiving palliative or hospice care, they often do not discuss spirituality with them.

Preferred Practice 20

- Develop and document a plan based on assessment of religious, spiritual, and existential concerns using a structured instrument and integrate the information obtained from the assessment into the palliative care plan.

Rationale

The NHPCO Standards Committee has developed guidelines for hospice programs, and according to these standards, spiritual concerns are to be addressed during the patient assessment.

Preferred Practice 21

- Provide information about the availability of spiritual care services and make spiritual care available either through organizational spiritual counseling or through the patient's own clergy relationships.

Rationale

Medicare regulations for hospice programs require a spiritual care counselor or other counselor on the interdisciplinary team.120 Additionally, the NHPCO Standards Committee has developed guidelines for hospice programs that state that clergy are to be part of, or at least available to, the interdisciplinary teams.

Preferred Practice 22

- Specialized palliative and hospice care teams should include spiritual care professionals appropriately trained and certified in palliative care.

Rationale

Specialized spiritual care often involves understanding and helping with specific theological beliefs and conflicts. It is ideally performed by persons with special training in this area, such as those trained as Clinical Pastoral Education chaplains.

BOX 1.2 (CONTINUED)

Preferred Practice 23

- Specialized palliative and hospice spiritual care professionals should build partnerships with community clergy, and provide education and counseling related to end-of-life care.

Rationale

Some patients prefer to use the local spiritual care counseling services of the religious entity to which they belong, however, local religious figures often do not have the appropriate training necessary for counseling palliative care patients and their families. The idea that spiritual care professionals with specialized skills in palliative care should serve as a community resource to local religious institutions is considered to be a "whole community" approach to end-of-life care that encourages communities to provide end-of-life information and support for patients and their families through religious congregations and educational programs. This approach is recommended by the Institute of Medicine.

Source: NQF (2006).

BOX 1.3 NASW STANDARDS FOR CULTURAL COMPETENCE

Standard 9. Cultural Competence

Social workers shall have, and shall continue to develop, specialized knowledge and understanding about history, traditions, values, and family systems as they relate to palliative and end of life care within different groups. Social workers shall be knowledgeable about, and act in accordance with, the *NASW Standards for Cultural Competence in Social Work Practice* (NASW, 2001).

Interpretation:

Social workers respect and integrate knowledge about how individuals and families are influenced by their ethnicity, culture, values, religion- and health-related beliefs, and economic situations. Social workers should understand systems of oppression and how these systems affect client access to, and utilization of, palliative and end of life care. Many cultures maintain their own values and traditions in the areas of palliative and end of life care.

BOX 1.3   (CONTINUED)

Culture influences individuals' and families' experience as well as the experience of the practitioner and institution. Social workers should consider culture in practice settings involving palliative and end of life care. Each cultural group has its own views about palliative and end of life practices and these need to be understood as they affect individuals' response to dying, death, illness, loss, and pain.

Social workers who understand how culture affects the illness and end of life experience of an individual and family will be better able to individualize care and intervene in the psychosocial impact of illness, pain, dying, and death. Therefore, social workers should be familiar with the practices and beliefs of the cultural groups with whom they practice to deliver culturally sensitive services.

Source: NASW (2004).)

care (p. 25). The *Code of Ethics of the National Association of Social Workers* (2008) and the CSWE *Educational Policy and Accreditation Standards* (2008; 2015a) also express the importance of understanding how religion and spirituality can shape human behavior and development and of respecting religious and spiritual beliefs that inform a patient's culture (CSWE, 2015b, CSWE, 2015c; Gilligan & Furness, 2006; Graff, 2007; Hodge et al., 2006). This includes the need for social workers to be mindful of their own belief systems and the implications for practice, particularly when a patient's beliefs are in conflict with those of the social worker. Social workers are also expected to consider a patient's religious and spiritual beliefs as sources of strength that inform interventions. Therefore, hospice social workers need to understand how spirituality may shape human behavior and be a source of strength, how spiritual diversity manifests in society and can enhance risk for discrimination, and how to build relationships that are spiritually sensitive to convey *spiritual* competence (NASW, 2008, 2015).

FACILITATING SPIRITUAL CARE

There is no guarantee that social workers will be able to fully utilize their expertise as members of interdisciplinary teams, but it is the responsibility of social workers to be prepared to do so. It takes collaboration for the collective strength of interdisciplinary teamwork to be realized (Goldsmith et al., 2010). Social workers are uniquely qualified to inform services that support patient psychosocial *and* spiritual well-being (Bliss & While, 2007; James, 2012; Lawson, 2007; Meier & Beresford, 2008; Monroe & DeLoach, 2004; Payne, 2009; Reese, 2011b, 2013). However, some researchers have noted that social workers have been "conspicuous by their absence" (Clausen, Kendall, Murray, Worth, Boyd, & Benton, 2005, p. 278; Stirling, 2007). Perhaps social workers are "not comfortable dealing with the spiritual dimensions of life" and so defer to interdisciplinary team members to take the lead (Puchalski et al., 2006, p. 408). Although Medicare requires a spiritual caregiver to be a member of the interdisciplinary team, all interdisciplinary team members can support patient access to quality spiritual care (Lawson, 2007). Social workers must be prepared to respond, given the risk for a patient's spiritual needs to go unmet. This is particularly important when spiritual suffering is evident and patient access to spiritual care is limited (Reese, 2013; Reith & Payne, 2009). However, social workers must be willing to communicate spiritual sensitivity and build spiritual competence to fully contribute during the short time patients receive care.

Chaplains as Essential Partners

Patients are likely to receive hospice care in their homes and may feel isolated from religious communities or be in need of spiritual support (Koenig, 2007). The need to be spiritually sensitive may be especially important for patients who are religious and/or report having more spiritual needs, including patients who are African American, Hispanic, older, female, single, lower income, and/or live in the South (Balboni, Vanderwerker, Block, Paulk, Lathan, Peteet, & Prigerson, 2007; Briggs & Rayle, 2005; Callahan, 2015; Canda & Furman, 1999, 2010; Gilligan & Furness, 2006; Hermann, 2007; Hodge, 2005a, 2011; Hodge et al., 2006; Modesto et al., 2006; Nelson-Becker & Canda, 2008). Spiritual needs can also emerge as part of the dying process. One way to facilitate spiritual care is to learn about the roles and responsibilities of other interdisciplinary team members who share in this responsibility (Goldsmith et al., 2010; Lawson, 2007; Meier & Beresford, 2008). Medicare-certified hospices are required to have a spiritual caregiver, like a board-certified chaplain

(Condition of Participation: Core Services, 2010; NHPCO, n.d., a). Although chaplains are usually theologically trained based on their individual religious affiliation, board-certified chaplains (BCCs) have additional training to serve patients from diverse backgrounds (Koenig, 2007; Puchalski et al., 2006).

Chaplains can seek certification through professional organizations like the Association of Professional Chaplains (APC, 2000, 2015a). The APC is the largest national chaplaincy organization, with approximately 4,000 members, and has worked to establish uniform professional standards across chaplaincy organizations (APC, 2004a; Koenig, 2007). The APC worked with five other professional chaplaincy organizations (representing more than 10,000 members) to establish the nationally recognized *Common Standards for Professional Chaplaincy* (APC, 2004a); *Common Code of Ethics for Chaplains, Pastoral Counselors, Pastoral Educators and Students* (APC, 2004b); and *Standards of Practice for Professional Chaplains in Hospice and Palliative Care* (APC, 2015b). To become a BCC, a candidate must have a graduate-level theological degree, religious endorsement through ordination or commission, completion of four units of clinical pastoral education (CPE), and demonstrated proficiency in 22 BCC competencies. One unit of CPE is 100 hours of education and 300 hours of supervised clinical experience (called a "residency"; APC, 2015a). A BCC must maintain his or her religious endorsement, complete annual continuing education, and have a peer review every fifth year. The APC also recognizes associated certified chaplains (ACCs), who have similar credentials but abridged CPE and continuing education requirements (Koenig, 2007).

Although chaplains and social workers have different educational backgrounds, they share similar values, ethics, and practices that inform patient-centered care (Koenig, 2007). For example, as described in the *Common Code of Ethics for Chaplains, Pastoral Counselors, Pastoral Educators and Students* (APC, 2004b):

> Spiritual Care Professionals are grounded in communities of faith and informed by professional education and training. They are called to nurture their personal health of mind, body and spirit and be responsible for their personal and professional conduct as they grow in their respect for all living beings and the natural environment. When Spiritual Care Professionals

behave in a manner congruent with the values of this code of ethics, they bring greater justice, compassion and healing to our world. Spiritual Care Professionals: affirm the dignity and value of each individual; respect the right of each faith group to hold to its values and traditions; advocate for professional accountability that protects the public and advances the profession; and respect the cultural, ethnic, gender, racial, sexual-orientation, and religious diversity of other professionals and those served and strive to eliminate discrimination.

(pp. 1–3)

Standards of Practice for Professional Chaplains in Hospice and Palliative Care (APC, 2015b) also clarifies the responsibilities of hospice chaplains, some of which are shared with hospice social workers, such as:

- Completing an assessment and determination of an individualized plan of care that contributes to the overall care of the patient that is measurable and documented.
- Participating in interdisciplinary teamwork and collaboration.
- Providing spiritual/religious resources, such as sacred texts, Shabbat candles, music, prayer rugs and rosaries.
- Offering or facilitating rituals, prayer and sacraments.
- Contributing in ethical issues, such as through a primary chaplaincy relationship, participation on an ethics committee or consultation team and/or participation on an institutional review board.
- Helping identify and interpret *cultures* and faith traditions that impact health-care practice and decisions.
- Educating and consulting with the health-care staff and the broader community.
- Building relationships with local faith communities and their leaders on behalf of the organization.
- Offering care and counsel to patients, their caregivers and staff regarding dynamic issues, including loss/grief, spiritual/religious/existential struggle, as well as strengths, opportunities for change and transformation, ethical decision making, and difficult communication or interpersonal dynamic situations.
- Facilitating difficult conversations including goals of care and advance care planning.

- Addressing signs and symptoms of non-physical pain and suffering.
- Providing leadership within the organization and within the broader field of chaplaincy.

(p. 6)

Since hospice organizations generally employ fewer chaplains who work part-time and/or serve in a volunteer capacity, they may need to rely more on interdisciplinary team members to help facilitate spiritual care (Reese, 2013). Social workers are among those team members who can help (Callahan, 2009b, 2012, 2013, 2015; Reese, 2001, 2011a, 2011b, 2013; Reese & Brown, 1997; Reese & Raymer, 2004; Reese et al., 2006). In a survey by Wittenberg-Lyles et al. (2008), the authors found that the majority of chaplains (63 percent) reported having a close working relationship with social workers and that half of these chaplains (50 percent) received the most support from social workers compared with other team members. Support might include joint visits, allowing social workers to learn more about chaplains through direct observation (Koenig, 2007; Meier & Beresford, 2008). Social workers may also need to educate patients about the role of chaplains and engage in spiritual assessment to inform referral (Koenig, 2007). Therefore, in supporting chaplains, social workers can facilitate patient access to spiritual care and develop their own capacity to provide spiritual care relative to professional expertise and patient needs.

CONCLUSION

Given the potential for social workers to be in situations in which spiritual issues emerge, they need the spiritual competence to operate in a manner that patients experience as spiritually sensitive (Reese, 2013). Spiritual competence is a more specific form of cultural competence (Hodge & Bushfield, 2006; Hodge et al., 2006). Spiritual competence requires social workers to understand how spirituality may shape human behavior and be a source of strength, how spiritual diversity manifests in society and can enhance risk for discrimination, and how to build relationships that are spiritually sensitive (NASW, 2008, 2015). To be spiritually sensitive, hospice social workers can utilize generalist practice skills to cultivate a therapeutic relationship that has the potential to enhance life meaning. Hospice social workers also need to be able to recognize a patient's spiritual needs, spiritual suffering, and spiritual resources. A referral to a spiritual caregiver may be required for follow-up, although the hospice social worker should be prepared to use advanced generalist and/or clinical practice skills to address a patient's spiritual needs, if necessary. The work of Hodge (2011) and associates (Hodge & Bushfield, 2006; Hodge et al., 2006) suggests the building of spiritual competence is a continuous process that involves an awareness of the individual's own worldview and assumptions, empathic understanding of a patient's worldview, and interventions that are sensitive to a patient's worldview. Therefore, hospice social workers need to be spiritually sensitive and prepared to facilitate patient access to timely spiritual care by referral, if not directly. Such preparedness is necessary in case a patient expresses an urgent need for spiritual care and/or refuses a referral to a formal spiritual-care provider.

Despite the need for hospice social workers to facilitate patient access to spiritual care, concern about addressing the complex nature of spirituality is understandable. BCCs are still needed in the professional role of spiritual caregiver. However, hospice social workers are also responsible for employing generalist skills to deliver care that is spiritually sensitive and to collaborate with others to spiritually support patients. Hospice social workers may need to enhance spiritual competence, particularly to draw from advanced generalist or clinical skills for the direct provision of spiritual care. Continuing education can sharpen awareness of how spirituality manifests in practice and how to spiritually support patients within professional boundaries. Practice and supervision can further help ensure patients experience hospice social work as spiritually sensitive. The actual experience of spiritual sensitivity can only be validated through patient assessment and treatment evaluation. Regardless, hospice social workers can strive to build spiritual competence as practitioner-learners on interdisciplinary teams. This enhances the ability of hospice social workers to both communicate in a spiritually sensitive manner with patients and create spiritually sensitive conditions on interdisciplinary teams and in the larger treatment environment (Canda & Furman, 1999, 2010). In the process of being champions of spiritual care, hospice social workers can enhance the overall quality of hospice care and, most importantly, the quality of life for patients facing terminal illness. The next chapter will initiate this process by defining spirituality and the importance of understanding how patients and their families define spirituality to inform respect for spiritual diversity.

2

Spiritual Diversity

IT CAN BE DIFFICULT TO understand the meaning of spirituality. Although most research has been conducted in the field of nursing, challenges in defining spirituality have emerged in research across disciplines (Henery, 2003a; Pike, 2011; Sinclair, Pereira, & Raffin, 2006). Conceptual ambiguity is also reflected in research limitations such as cultural bias in instrumentation and study population (Sinclair et al., 2006). Understanding spiritual diversity may help social workers tolerate some degree of conceptual ambiguity and at the same time help to clarify how spirituality informs practice, education, and research (Edwards et al., 2010; Henery, 2003a; Hodge & McGrew, 2005; Swinton & Pattison, 2010; Van der Steen et al., 2009; Sinclair et al., 2006). A patient's experience of spirituality can inform and be informed by the provision of hospice social work (Holloway et al., 2011; Pike, 2011). More specifically, therapeutic relationships provide a context through which a patient's experience of spirituality may enhance life meaning. This chapter will explore different definitions of spirituality to inspire respect for spiritual diversity and a foundation for the healing effects of relational spirituality.

EXPERIENCING SPIRITUALITY THROUGH RELATIONSHIPS

Academic literature across disciplines has often described spirituality as a transcendent connection within the self and/or with something outside the self, such as other people, the environment, or a divine higher power (Canda & Furman, 1999, 2010; Gijsberts et al., 2011; Hodge & McGrew, 2005;

Krieglstein, 2006; Pesut, 2008a; Pesut, Fowler, Reimer-Kirkham, Taylor, & Sawatzky, 2009; Reese, 2013; Vachon, Fillion, & Achille, 2009). Relationships can channel energy that enables survival. Relationships can push people to transcend perceived limits and therefore have the potential to be life enhancing (Canda & Furman, 1999, 2010; Gijsberts et al., 2011; Sulmasy, 2009). Spirituality may involve relationships that paradoxically lead to the experience of going beyond the self, described as transcendence (Gijsberts et al., 2011; Reese, 2013; Swinton & Pattison, 2010). Based on this perspective, all people are spiritual beings, as all people are in relationships that spark a dynamic process of self-actualization needed to operate in the world (Gijsberts et al., 2011; Krieglstein, 2006; Sulmasy, 2009; Swinton & Pattison, 2010).

Spirituality is also considered a universal, dynamic search for meaning. Although all people need to experience life meaning, what is considered meaningful is self-defined, for it is in relation to individual beliefs, priorities, and interpretation of experiences (Canda & Furman, 1999, 2010; Gijsberts et al., 2011; Krieglstein, 2006; Pesut et al., 2009; Reese, 2013). This means the experience of spirituality involves psychosocial processes, but a spiritual experience may be outside one's ability to observe and communicate. Religious worship may be meaningful for some but alienating for others (Hodge & McGrew, 2005; Krieglstein, 2006; Reese, 2013; Schneiders, 2003). Spirituality could manifest as an experience of deep peace while meditating alone or in service to others (Krieglstein, 2006). Therefore, a variety of contextual factors can facilitate a spiritually transcendent, meaningful connection. It is the premise of this book that hospice social workers can engage with patients in a therapeutic relationship that enhances life meaning. The experience of spirituality gained through meaningful relationships is defined as relational spirituality.

A STUDY IN CONTRASTS

Beyond considering the relational aspects of spirituality, many facets of spirituality defy clarification. It is also misleading to suggest that every patient could relate to or understand the experience of spirituality as being informed by relationships. Although the idea of relational spirituality can provide a foundation for hospice social work, spiritual sensitivity necessitates hospice social workers appreciate spiritual diversity. To help, a review

of conceptual contradictions follows that demonstrates how spirituality could mean different things to different people. Relying on a patient's
understanding of spirituality to inform the context of care encourages hospice social workers to assume a position of cultural humility. Ultimately,
hospice social workers need the capacity to tolerate some ambiguity while
discerning a patient's worldview and creating conditions that a patient
experiences as spiritually supportive. It is this ability of hospice social workers to accept a patient's definition of spirituality that provides a necessary
foundation for being spiritually sensitive. In this relational process, spiritually sensitive hospice social work may emerge as a spiritual quality of care
that is life enhancing for patients and, potentially, hospice social workers.

Ineffable Versus Definable

Scholars have struggled with conceptual inconsistencies and contradictions in trying to define spirituality (Sinclair et al., 2006; Swinton & Pattison, 2010; Van der Steen et al., 2009). Some have said that ambiguity
allows for broader application across populations (Holloway et al., 2011).
Vachon et al. (2009) conducted a qualitative thematic analysis of pallia-
tive- and hospice- care research in effort to develop an integrated definition
of spirituality. They found that (1) meaning and purpose in life, (2) self-
transcendence, (3) transcendence with a higher being, (4) feelings of communion and mutuality, (5) beliefs and faith, (6) hope, (7) attitude toward
death, (8) appreciation of life, (9) reflection upon fundamental values, and
(10) the developmental nature of spirituality and (11) its conscious aspect
were all associated with spirituality at the end of life. In a follow-up study,
Gijsberts et al. (2011) found that the experience of meaning and purpose in
life was the only aspect of spirituality that was consistently reported in the
literature. They suggested that Vachon et al. did not control for conceptual
overlap. For example, "beliefs and faith" and "self-transcendence" were said
to be inclusive of "faith in self." Vachon et al. did not identify a distinctly
spiritual state either. "Feelings of communion and mutuality," "attitude
toward death," and an "appreciation of life" could be indicative of a psychological rather than a spiritual state (Koenig, 2008). The same could be
said for the "conscious aspect," which may be considered more of a physical
or cognitive state than a spiritual state. Gijsberts et al. suggested another
approach was needed to clearly define spirituality as a distinct construct.

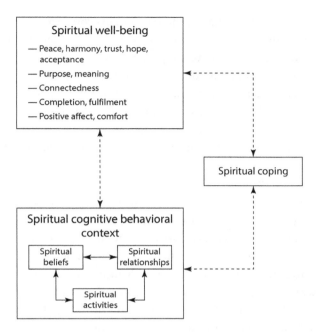

FIGURE 2.1   A model for the conceptualization of spirituality at the end of life.
Source: Gijsberts et al. (2011), p. 857.

Gijsberts et al. (2011) wondered whether some aspects of spirituality were more important or were experienced more often than others. The authors responded by developing a conceptual model of spirituality based on analyzing instruments used to measure spirituality at the end of life. As seen in figure 2.1, this model suggests that spiritual well-being, spiritual cognitive-behavioral context (including spiritual beliefs, spiritual activities, and spiritual relationships), spiritual coping, and the associations among them define spirituality. Although the authors were trying to identify discrete concepts, distinctions between these concepts still relied on the elusive definition of spirituality. The authors used spirituality to define itself in combination with other concepts that partially rely on the definition of spirituality to be fully understood. Furthermore, Gijsberts et al. did not explain how characteristics of spiritual well-being (or coping) could be distinguished from psychological well-being (or coping). The model also suggests that spirituality requires a particular cognitive-behavioral context without clarifying what that would be. Perhaps contextual factors, such as the quality of significant relationships or the atmosphere of the environment, would be more likely to support the experience of spirituality. The authors did not identify whether a particular level of cognitive capacity was necessary to experience spirituality or recognize the experience of spirituality. Although reliance on instruments implied a belief spirituality could be measured, Gijsberts et al.'s conceptualization of spirituality still seemed rather unclear and more an accurate reflection of biopsychosocial processes.

CONCLUSION

Despite efforts toward integration, conceptual ambiguity has been challenging to reconcile. Upon closer examination, the concept of spirituality has been either broadly inclusive or narrow in scope, while still failing to recognize the potential fluidity of spirituality as a state of being or stage of development (Bregman, 2006; Reese, 2013; Swinton & Pattison, 2010). Both approaches validate a singular, static way of defining spirituality that may lead to false ideas about what spirituality means for hospice patients. This either-or approach can also lead to assumptions that one person with a particular worldview is more spiritual than another person with a different worldview (Senreich, 2013). Hence, one needs to be cautious and not define spirituality too narrowly (Bregman, 2006). Perhaps a single definition may not be feasible (Holloway et al., 2011; MacConville, 2006; Van der Steen et al., 2009). It could be that a degree of ambiguity is good for hospice social workers, for it requires them to rely more on patients to define spirituality for themselves (Holloway et al., 2011).

Individual Versus Universal

Spirituality has been associated with a sense of purpose that includes the inspiration to forge meaningful connections, some of which facilitate transcendence. It has been suggested that spirituality is woven into all aspects of life and thus emerges through mystical as well as mundane experiences (Broughton, 2006). As such, any person has the potential to experience spirituality, which makes this type of experience universal (Canda, 1999; Krieglstein, 2006; Sulmasy, 2009). Although spirituality is considered to be a natural aspect of being human, what makes something spiritual is relative to one's subjective experience. This hinges on the capacity to reflect upon an experience and identify it as being spiritual. However, this may not be possible for people with a limited ability to self-reflect. Confusion, impaired thoughts, and semiconscious states can all be associated with the dying process (Van der Steen et al., 2009). Does this mean that hospice patients cease to be spiritual beings or do not have spiritual experiences during the dying process? Another challenge in assuming that spirituality is a universal experience is the reference point used to define a spiritual experience.

The majority of research about spirituality, including palliative- and hospice-care research, relies on samples of the general population rather than hospice patients (Hodge & McGrew, 2005; Pike, 2011; Swinton & Pattison, 2010). These results are further limited by small sample sizes and low response rates (Draper, 2011; Hodge & McGrew, 2005). Studies about spirituality may further attract people particularly interested in sharing their own worldviews, which may not reflect the experience of people who view spirituality as a private matter or who are not as spiritually articulate (Hodge & McGrew, 2005). Studies that include people from different religious traditions, depending on sampling method, may not be generalizable either. Their views may not be congruent with religious dictates or beliefs of those in a similar religious tradition regardless of whether that person is in hospice care or not. Even within hospice care, what professionals think patients experience spiritually may not be congruent with what patients actually experience (McSherry et al., 2004). Hence, research that attempts to describe the spirituality of hospice patients *for* hospice patients may not represent what each individual patient understands spirituality to be.

Limits in applying research results to hospice patients extend beyond the risk of sampling bias and low response rate. The types of instruments used in these studies are also a product of particular ideas about what defines spirituality. Efforts to capture a universal experience of spirituality may still fail to reflect an individual's experience. Measurement instruments that are the product of a particular theory can also yield results that are likely to be interpreted within the same theoretical framework. Theoretical models that define spirituality too broadly may include unrelated biopsychosocial factors that inaccurately inform measurements. Conversely, measurements may include questions that reflect a particular experience of spirituality that is too narrow in scope (Gijsberts et al., 2011). Hodge (2007a) references a measure by Whitfield (1984) that associates sexual gratification with having a spiritual experience. Those spiritually committed to abstinence would get a lower score and would be considered less spiritual. Hence, this "universal" definition of spirituality may be operationalized in a way that fails to be truly inclusive of those who view themselves as spiritual and/or religious.

CONCLUSION

To understand the experience of hospice patients, research must include them. In addition, what defines a spiritual experience has traditionally been associated with positive emotional descriptors. Pesut (2008b) says that this tends to "pathologize the basic human experience of suffering and marginalize those most vulnerable in society" (p. 167). So, the discourse on spirituality needs to be more inclusive of diverse experiences of spirituality, even though some of these experiences may seem to be negative (Edwards et al., 2010; Swinton & Pattison, 2010). One of the challenges is to recognize and use the language of spirituality as suggested by patients, rather than to impose the language of one's own spirituality on patients (Swinton & Pattison, 2010; Pesut, 2008b). This, of course, assumes that a patient operates from a spiritual worldview. A patient's internal state may not be known by a hospice social worker, particularly if the patient is unable to understand or articulate it (Senreich, 2013). In these cases, perhaps, those who know the patient best may provide a hospice social worker guidance in determining what is congruent with a patient's worldview.

Spiritual Versus Religious

Similar to the idea of being "spiritual but not religious," the conceptual of spirituality as being separate from religion has been set forth by some scholars, while others have described spirituality and religion as being related if not identical (Hodge & McGrew, 2005; Pesut et al., 2009; Sulmasy, 2009). As related constructs, religion and spirituality inform each other. The practice of religion can be one of many ways if not *the* way people experience spirituality (Stanworth, 2006; Sulmasy, 2009; Vachon et al., 2009). Even though the conceptual relationship between spirituality and religion is complex, spirituality and religion have increasingly been considered distinct concepts in palliative- and hospice-care research (Garces-Foley, 2006; Sulmasy, 2009; Vachon et al., 2009; Walter, 2002). This trend has included assertions that being spiritual is more desirable than, if not superior to, being religious (Adams, 2006; Henery, 2003a; Hodge & McGrew, 2005; Garces-Foley, 2006; Koenig, 2008).

There are many definitions associated with religion (Hodge & McGrew, 2005), although religion is generally described as "an organized faith system, beliefs, worship, religious rituals, and relationship with a divine being" (Vachon et al., 2009, p. 53). More specifically, according to Henery (2003), religion is a "communal phenomenon" (p. 1111) that Hodge & McGrew (2005) say occurs in a "communal setting" (p. 17) in which religious beliefs are organized and practiced. Goddard (1995) further says that "religion exemplifies a particular value and belief system and provides an ethical-moral code, or framework, for behaviour" in daily life but is shaped by "contemporary cultural values and personal philosophies" (pp. 809–810). Religion is therefore a "multi-faceted phenomenon" that is shaped by a social and historical context (Van Hook & Rivera, 2004, p. 234). Koenig (2008) confirms that religion is "easier to define and measure" as a shared tradition with particular religious beliefs like those associated with life after death and religious practices like prayer alone or in community (n.p.).

Sulmasy (2009) describes spirituality as being both broadly inclusive and individually specific. Spirituality is considered more inclusive than religion in that all people engage in questions of transcendence, regardless of religious affiliation. Spirituality is also viewed as being more individualized than religion, in that one's relationship with the transcendent is ultimately personal. According to Sulmasy, there are "as many spiritualities as there are individuals" (p. 1635), which Kellehear (2000) says reflects one's evolving "human need to transcend, to go beyond the immediacy of suffering and to find meaning in that experience" (p. 153). Belcher and Griffiths (2005) conclude that "the definition of spirituality . . . [is] the innate human yearning for meaning through intra-, inter-, and transpersonal connectedness" (p. 272). Since spirituality is "defined by the universal search for meaning, connectedness, energy, and transcendence," Pesut (2008a) says it is "no longer rooted within religion" (p. 98). As such, Koenig (2008) recognizes that spirituality is "difficult to define and quantify" (n.p.).

CONCLUSION

Even though a distinction has been made between spirituality and religion, hospice patients might not be quite as clear. McSherry et al. (2004) conducted a qualitative study to compare how hospice patients and nurses defined spirituality and found that patients and nurses defined spirituality differently. In fact, the patients in this study were unclear about the meaning of spirituality. They did consider spirituality to be synonymous with religion, but this relationship seemed to be relative to the patient's religious affiliation. The authors suggested that these patients did not adhere to a single, universal definition of spirituality, so caution needed to be used in addressing spirituality with patients. They also said the same approach might not apply with all patients given variation in the experience of spirituality even among patients with the same religious affiliation. Hence, it is best to solicit information about a patient's understanding of spirituality and the potential role of religion rather than relying on preconceived notions.

Individual Versus Relational

Spirituality has been considered a highly individualistic, humanistic endeavor (Canda, 1999). Sulmasy (2009) describes these aspects of spirituality "as the ways in which a person habitually conducts his or her life in relationship to the question of transcendence . . . each relationship with the transcendent will always be unique and spirituality ultimately personal" (p. 1635). As previously stated, Sulmasy concludes there are "as many spiritualities as there are individuals" (p. 1635), which is echoed by Krieglstein (2006), who says there are "different types of spirituality" (p. 21). Krieglstein goes on to suggest that "relational spirituality" is a type of spirituality indicated by the experience of spirituality through relationships, but the author does not describe how these relationships may unfold (p. 26). The spiritual importance of relationships is also referenced by MacConville (2006), who states that "for some people, their spirituality or their connection may be centred on relationships; this may be a relationship with God, although religious practice may not form part of that relationship" (p. 145).

How spiritually informs life meaning may be "individualistic," but not the "individual search for meaning" (MacConville, 2006, p. 145). There may be different ways to search for life meaning, but generally all people need to experience meaning in life. Relationships may be one way to experience life meaning and can be an expression of spirituality. Spirituality may be considered a connection with the self, others, the environment, or a higher power. This means spirituality can be informed by a relationship even if that relationship is with the self as part of, for example, self-care or contemplation. Social context helps to inform what is meaningful, as individual perceptions are influenced by significant others. Likewise, Edwards et al. (2010) found in a systemic review of palliative-care research that spirituality is "inherently relational" and "connections with family and significant others, rather than just meaning making, appears [to be] the most important dimension of spirituality." They also said that, "patients most often found meaning in relationships" (p. 764).

Vachon et al. (2009) suggest that by going deep within and/or reaching outside the self, relationships can be a means of transcendence. Relationships that support the experience of transcendence would be considered those that enhance life meaning, although this process of relating may necessitate the experience of both positive and negative emotions. It is not clear whether all people are willing to seek the experience of transcendence or have the capacity to cultivate relationships that facilitate such transcendence. As detailed by the authors, transcendence:

> Involves a profound self-reflection and a will to go beyond the self in accomplishing actions and living according to one's profound values . . . It also implies a deep faith in the self (and in one's unique purpose in life), as well as faith in others in mutual relationships that allows one to appreciate the precious value of life. Transcendence with a Higher Being also characterizes the spiritual experience and is characterized by a feeling of connection and mutuality with a higher power, which allows one to give meaning to life and death.
>
> (p. 56)

Hence, Vachon et al. suggest that transcendence is a transitory state that entails seeking meaningful connections with the self, others, and/or God or a higher power. Transcendence is further contingent upon what is valued and may be in response to a desire to cultivate what is valued in life. Hospice patients may seek interpersonal relationships that help them transcend suffering in making peace with the past and present and finding hope in the future, although the process of cultivating a deep intrapersonal connection with the self may also allow for such transcendence.

Ellison (1983) developed a vertical-horizontal approach that also suggests relational aspects of spirituality. These relational aspects are indicated

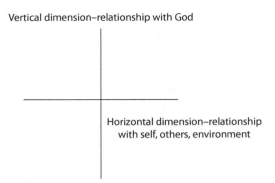

Vertical dimension–relationship with God

Horizontal dimension–relationship
with self, others, environment

FIGURE 2.2   Vertical-horizontal approach.
Source: Carroll (2001).

by two intersecting lines that represent two means of connection, like in the image by Carroll (2001) in figure 2.2. Since this model includes a divine deity, it would only apply to patients with a particular worldview (like other definitions of spirituality). The vertical dimension would be shaped by ideas about a divine entity as well as moral or ethical values. The horizontal dimension consists of a clearer psychosocial component. As suggested by the authors, there is a degree of interaction that occurs between the vertical and horizontal dimensions, so for example, beliefs about one's relationship with the divine on the vertical dimension may inform how to engage in relationships with others and the environment on the horizontal dimension (Carroll, 2001; Ellison, 1983).

CONCLUSION

Relationships that lead to transcendence can help define spirituality. At a root level, a transcendent connection requires a desire to be known (Pesut, 2008b). Transcendence can evoke experiences that push the bounds of existence. Models serve to provide a simple example of processes that may unfold, but in some respects what lends power to the experience of transcendence is the fact that the magnitude of the experience pales in comparison when language seeks to contain it (Pesut, 2008b). One means of recourse is to explore the contextual factors that emerge as part of the spiritual experience when caring for patients. Coupled with the previously mentioned research, the experience of understanding a patient's spiritual perspective and being comfortable with one's own spirituality can provide essential information for the provision of patient-centered, spiritually sensitive hospice social work.

STYMIED BY SOCIAL CONSTRUCTION

Given the limits of research and breadth of human diversity, it is impossible to fully describe what spirituality means. Religious studies scholars consider spirituality to be a part of religion. For some patients, however, the experience of spirituality may be a secular truth (Bell, 2006; Garces-Foley, 2006). Wong and Vinsky (2009) charged that "Euro-Christian ethnocentrism and individualism" (p. 1343) have rendered invisible the experiences of people with different worldviews. This limits insight into the spiritual strengths of persons outside those traditions (Holloway et al., 2011). Even if dominant research on spirituality reflects cultural hegemony, this perspective also risks implying homogeneity of minority views (McSherry et al., 2004). In fact, the meaning of spirituality may vary widely among people in culturally similar Western countries like the United States compared with a more secular United Kingdom and among liberal to conservative Christians within the same religious denomination (Garces-Foley, 2006; Hodge, 2007a; McSherry et al., 2004; Pesut, 2008b).

Defining spiritual diversity has been challenging even for religious studies scholars (Garces-Foley, 2006; Pesut, 2008a). According to Garces-Foley (2006), religious studies scholars have viewed "spirituality as a particular cultural expression of religion rather than a universal dimension of human life and have tried to understand the many different meanings people in Western societies attribute to spirituality" (p. 127). Nevertheless, research on spirituality has largely been conducted by scholars in Western societies (Garces-Foley, 2006; Sinclair et al., 2006; Stanworth, 2006; Walter, 2002; Wong & Vinsky, 2009) from a Christian perspective (Garces-Foley, 2006; McSherry et al., 2004; Pike, 2011; Walter, 2002; Ward, 2005; Wong & Vinsky, 2009). Religious studies scholars have also focused on the experience of people in Western societies, a trend seen in research on spirituality across disciplines (Sinclair et al., 2006). Therefore, as a cultural artifact, research on spirituality reflects the dominant culture in how it is measured and, potentially, experienced by those involved in such research.

Negotiating Contextual Boundaries

To build conceptual clarity, it makes sense to treat spirituality like a quantifiable concept (Henery, 2003a; Pesut, 2008b). Conceptual models, like those by Gijsberts et al. (2011) and Ellison (1983), include "parts, components and vertical and horizontal dimensions" that suggest spirituality is "ready for measurement, insertion, replacement and manipulation" (Henery, 2003a, p. 555). As previously noted, however, such reductionism may exclude people with different experiences of spirituality. This is true even with what seems to be a broadly inclusive definition of spirituality. Some people may experience spirituality in a way that, for example, extends beyond common language or comprehension (Egan et al., 2011; Pesut, 2008a; Swinton & Pattison, 2010). As described by Stanworth (2006), "Life is larger than language and there is no tidy encapsulation of spirituality that does not artificially foreclose enquiry and meaning" (p. 28). In some cases, metaphors and stories are needed to "make real for us what cannot otherwise be said" (p. 27).

Multiple sources of information must be used to define spirituality, which Stanworth (2006) says, "Prevents us from approaching spirituality as an exclusively Western, individualistic, and post-Enlightenment search for meaning and purpose" (p. 28). Swinton and Pattison (2010) agree that "multiple definitions may be indicative of the necessity and the flexibility of the term to meet particular needs that would otherwise go unmet" (p. 231). A lack of conceptual clarity does not make it any less significant (Swinton & Pattison, 2010). Properly understood, an inclusive definition of spirituality may still be more conceptually accurate, provided the experience of spirituality is an evolving state relative to each person's life trajectory. Conversations about spirituality also provide "a way of naming absences and recognizing gaps in healthcare provision" (Swinton & Pattison, 2010, p. 226). Hospice social workers are charged with shared responsibility for minimizing patient suffering, so conversations about a patient's spirituality may help that patient find meaning and ultimately transcend the experience of spiritual suffering (Edwards et al., 2010; Pike, 2011).

Therefore, a review of the literature would suggest that what makes something spiritual is defined differently relative to each person and the context within which that person operates (Egan et al., 2011; Henery, 2003a; McSherry et al., 2004; Pike, 2011; Swinton & Pattison, 2010;

Takahashi & Ide, 2003). This means spirituality is considered a social construct; however, it does not mean that spirituality is *only* a social construct (Swinton & Pattison, 2010). While it is not appropriate to rely solely on a definition that is too broad or too narrow in scope, it is appropriate to make efforts to understand and accommodate various definitions of spirituality (Pesut, 2008b). In this respect, it is important for hospice social workers to engage in conversations with patients about what gives life meaning and sustains resilience (Pike, 2011; Swinton & Pattison, 2010). The experience of spirituality may be different for hospice patients compared with the general population and may likewise change over time as conditions change. This necessitates ongoing efforts to determine whether patient spirituality has implications for the delivery of hospice social work (Pesut, 2008b).

A Return to Relationship

There are many reasons for hospice social workers to address spirituality with patients (see table 2.1). Among the most profound reasons is to understand a patient's spiritual needs, given the potential for spiritual suffering (Bynum et al., 2016; Gijsberts et al, 2011; National Hospice and Palliative Care Organization, 2014, 2015b; Peteet & Balboni, 2013; Reese, 2013; Reith & Payne, 2009). In the process of collaborating with patients, hospice social workers need to rely on current research to inform practice. However, studies evaluating spiritual care are few in number and have conceptual and measurement issues and limited samples (Draper, 2011; Edwards et al., 2010; Hodge & McGrew, 2005; McSherry et al., 2004; Pike, 2011; Swinton & Pattison, 2010). One concern is reliance on samples from the general population or health-care professionals to make inferences about how hospice patients define spirituality (Edwards et al., 2010; McSherry et al., 2004; Pike, 2011). Hospice social workers need to make a concerted effort to understand how patients define spirituality and whether patients' experience of spirituality changes throughout the progression of illness. Research in this area has not advanced enough to include a review of longitudinal research, but there is some research specific to hospice patients that lends insight into their experiences.

Draper (2011) conducted a review of empirical research on spirituality and health care published between 2005 and 2011. The author reported that there were 15 empirical studies that incorporated samples of patients, with

TABLE 2.1   Reasons to Address Spirituality

TYPE	EXPLANATION
Patient expectations	Patient expresses a spiritual and/or religious worldview, reports a religious affiliation, and solicits spiritual support.
Spiritual needs	Patient relies on spiritual resources, expresses a desire for spiritual resources (has limited access to spiritual support), and reflects signs of spiritual suffering.
Developmentally appropriate	The dying process is considered a developmental stage of life with associated needs, such as the need to process emotional response to loss.
Change in medical status	First diagnosis, symptoms (remission/active dying), medication side effects, and duration (acute/chronic).
Component of holistic care	The tradition of hospice is to provide biopsychosocial-spiritual care that supports the collective needs of patients and their caregivers.
Mandated by accrediting organizations	The Joint Commission authorizes hospice providers for Medicare reimbursement.
Supported by professional organizations	Professional organizations across disciplines have recognized the importance of respect for patient spirituality. This includes social work organizations such as the National Association of Social Workers (NASW), Council on Social Work Education (CSWE), Society for Spirituality and Social Work (SSSW), and the North American Association of Christians in Social Work (NACSW).
Therapeutic effects	Spiritual resources, such as positive religious coping by maintaining faith through prayer and reconciliation, have the potential to enhance life quality.

Sources: Callahan, 2008, 2009a, 2009b, 2016; Canda & Furman, 1999, 2010; Carson & Koenig, 2004; CSWE, 2008, 2015a, 2015b, 2015c; Cunningham, 2012; Derezotes, 2006; Hermann, 2007; Hodge, 2003; Hodge & Bushfield, 2006; Horton-Parker & Fawcett, 2010; Joint Commission, 2016; Knight & von Gunten, 2004c; Koenig, 2007, 2008; Lee, Ng, Leung, & Chan, 2009; Mathews, 2009; Mitchell, Bennett, & Manfrin-Ledet, 2006; Murray, Kendall, Boyd, Worth, & Benton, 2004; Murray, Kendall, Grant, Boyd, Barclay, & Sheikh, 2007; NACSW, 2008; NASW, 2001, 2004, 2008, 2015; Pargament, 2007; Puchalski, 2006; Reese, 2013; SSSW, n.d.; Taylor, 2007.

11 studies being qualitative. Only three of those studies had a sample size of at least 20. The majority of research was on the spiritual needs of hospice patients and/or receiving palliative care. The author found that research was beginning to be more inclusive of people from Eastern cultures as well as nonreligious people. In particular, there were two studies that included a survey with 88 participants (Smith-Stoner, 2007) and a qualitative study with 11 participants (Creel, 2007) that focused on the experience of nonreligious patients. The authors found that these patients wanted professionals to respect their beliefs. Based on Smith-Stoner (2007), this included a preference for evidence-based interventions with the option for physician-assisted suicide and no reference to God or an offering of prayer. Participants further expressed a desire to find meaning in life and to experience connections with family, friends, and the natural world.

Edwards et al. (2010) conducted a systematic literature review and found that out of the 19 qualitative studies on spirituality and palliative care published between 2001 and 2009, 11 were on the experiences of patients. These studies included a total of 178 patients. The majority of patients had cancer and were elderly, white, and Judeo-Christian. The authors further analyzed these studies to determine how patients defined spirituality. Edwards et al. found that these patients had trouble defining spirituality but often referred to significant relationships to describe their experience of spirituality. Spirituality was also expressed through the telling of life-affirming stories that reflected gratitude and a reverence for life. Finally, spirituality was described as being informed by hope, meaning, and purpose in life that extended to an afterlife. The authors concluded that relationships or connections, followed by one's pride in accomplishments, informed life meaning. These data further suggested that spirituality was not tied to religion but was considered to be something larger than life and thus difficult to define.

The findings of Draper (2011) and Edwards et al. (2010) lend support to the definition of spirituality as being the product of a patient's understanding of what spirituality is within the context of one's experience. These findings further support the idea of relational spirituality (Krieglstein, 2006; MacConville, 2006). If relationships provide a foundation for a patient's experience of spirituality, then it seems that the type of therapeutic relationship a social worker builds with a patient may have spiritual implications as well. This is important, for the helping relationship is the primary mode of service delivery for hospice social workers. Relationship building allows a hospice social worker to move from stranger to ally. It is through relationship that a hospice social worker comes to understand how a patient perceives the world. Hence, the helping relationship provides the most immediate opportunity for hospice social workers to understand the spirituality of patients. Spiritual sensitivity is required for the spirituality of patients to come into focus and to serve as a resource for care.

CONCLUSION

Striving for a universal definition of spirituality may be futile. Misunderstandings can flourish when the definition of spirituality is based on a dubious conceptual and empirical foundation (Hodge, 2007a). This can be seen in research, where a contentious divide between spirituality and religion has emerged. Assumptions about what spirituality means for patients based on majority views may fail to recognize spiritual diversity. Perhaps the best way to understand a patient's definition of spirituality is to bear witness to one's spirituality through the context of the therapeutic relationship (MacConville, 2006). "Shared by analogies of experience across cultural and religious backgrounds," but not necessarily anchored in formal religion, spirituality may provide a whole new way of seeing a patient and facilitating the healing process (Stanworth, 2006, p. 27). This style of engagement may be a resource for the delivery of spiritually sensitive hospice social work, but additional concepts must be reviewed in the remainder of this book to realize this potential. In the end, it is essential for hospice social workers to tolerate some degree of ambiguity when defining spirituality, because a patient's understanding of spirituality may evolve throughout the dying process. Ongoing assessment is required for clarification that informs further action even if such action is simply to be a companion on the journey until death. The next chapter will explore spiritual needs as reported by patients and what factors might contribute to patients' needs as part of the dying process.

3

Spiritual Needs

GROWTH CAN OCCUR IN RESPONSE to life transitions marked by birth, childhood, adolescence, adulthood, and old age. The dying process may be considered another life transition with universal challenges and those unique to each person. This developmental perspective does not suggest a patient must achieve specific goals or tasks to experience a good death. Life quality associated with the dying process is shaped by multiple factors like a patient's age and duration of illness. The delivery of hospice care is an effort to maintain life quality of both patient and caregiver. Although it is not possible to fully comprehend what it is like to go through the dying process, hospice social workers can develop valuable insights into the developmental challenges and subsequent needs of those who are dying (Prince-Paul, 2008). With this knowledge, hospice social workers can help patients grow as they confront their mortality (Reese, 2013; Reith & Payne, 2008). This chapter describes common spiritual needs and unique factors that can shape the experience of dying, giving hospice social workers better understanding of this natural and yet extraordinary part of life (Byock, 1996; Lamers, 2014).

PRESERVING PERSONHOOD

The dying process is the ultimate expression of one's humanity. However humbling reduced capacity may be, this process does not have to involve the loss of personhood. From a Western perspective, personhood is an individual expression of one's uniqueness (Hermann, 2001; Wright, 2002). Hospice care is designed to honor one's personhood throughout the dying process. This involves recognizing what defines a person and potential needs that person has. As described by Byock (1996):

> Each person has a prominent physical dimension, a body, which is unique and yet has important features in common with the bodies of other people . . . Additionally, each person possesses an inherent temperament and distinctive characteristics, preferences, aversions, habits and quirks that contribute to their uniqueness . . . Persons possess beliefs (ranging from political to metaphysical), moral values, and a sense of meaning. Persons also do things and identify with what they have done or wish to do. The active aspect of self extends from the outermost layers to the deepest concentric core of the person: from "activities of daily living" and mundane chores, to routine work-related projects, civic affairs and the normal relationships of community life to work toward the most meaningful of one's aspirations and relations of the most intimate nature. Considered collectively, activities form the medium through which nearly all the dimensions of self are given shape and texture. They are the medium through which the rich, unique composition of personhood can emerge.
>
> (pp. 240–241)

Terminal illness can profoundly shape one's sense of personhood. Personhood may be overshadowed by the symptoms of disease and frailty that compromise a person's ability to engage in an active life (Allamani, 2007; Prince-Paul, 2008). The acquired status of "patient" can exacerbate social isolation (Hermann, 2001; Hills et al., 2005). Emotions like fear, depression, and anger can emerge in response to existential questions (Heyse-Moore, 1996; Hills et al., 2005). Thus, the dying process can lead to specific needs as well as unique challenges.

In the midst of challenges, the experience of death is an important part of life that is informed by and informs personhood. This makes the dying process more than a series of biological events. The dying process is a complex part of human development in which personhood evolves up to the point of death (Allamani, 2007; Byock, 1996; Hermann, 2001; Reese, 2013; Reith & Payne, 2008). Although this process is profoundly personal, death is also a universal experience. As further described by Eilberg (2006):

> Each encounter with another human being is unique, each person's life story a world of its own. Individuals bring their own life experiences, wisdom, and needs to each encounter. Thus, there can never be a map of the territory of dying: The territory is too complex and mysterious for charting. Yet, it is possible to offer a sketch of what one may find when working in the presence of death. Every stage of life has its own challenges and opportunities... People who know that death is near have characteristic feelings and needs and a particular set of developmental challenges to face. Sometimes the challenges may present possibilities for learning, growth, and healing, even at the end of life.
>
> (p. 158)

What makes a person unique shapes both life and death, but the human condition carries with it the potential for suffering. The dying process allows one to move "from feeling beaten down to opening up to life" (Allamani, 2007, p. 231). This experience of suffering provides an opportunity for growth that occurs within and/or through community (Allamani, 2007; Byock, 1996; Eilberg, 2006). Hospice social workers can be among those who help patients move from despair and brokenness to integrity and wholeness (Edwards et al., 2010).

DEFINING SPIRITUAL NEEDS

It is not unusual to "reach out to what is seen as true and valuable" when faced with terminal illness (Saunders, 1988, p. 30; Cornette, 2005). Spirituality is important if not essential for some patients in hospice care, and addressing spiritual needs is therefore "an integral developmental task for those who are dying" (Puchalski, 2001, p. 353; Gijsberts et al., 2011; Hills et al., 2005; Hodge & Horvath, 2011; Kellehear, 2000; Penman et al., 2013; Peteet & Balboni, 2013). In research studies, more than 80 to 90 percent of patients have reported spiritual needs (Gijsberts et al., 2011; Peteet & Balboni, 2013). The death of the flesh is the ultimate test of the spirit and may be experienced as deeply threatening no matter how spiritual one may be (Pesut, 2008). The dying process can lead to feelings of loss, hopelessness, and abandonment, as well as forgiveness, peace, and acceptance, all of which can have spiritual implications (Hills et al., 2005; Lukoff, n.d.). Likewise, spiritual beliefs and practices have the potential to enhance spiritual well-being (Gijsberts et al., 2011; Hills et al., 2005). Therefore, addressing spiritual needs is one way to respond to the challenges of death (Dobratz, 2005; Edwards et al., 2010; Glasper, 2011; Kellehear, 2000; Murray, Kendall, Boyd, Worth, & Benton, 2004; Okon, 2005; Wright, 2002).

Spiritual needs are associated with beliefs and practices that may or may not involve religion but allow a person to connect with what is valued and gives life meaning (Dobratz, 2005; Glasper, 2011; Kellehear, 2000; Murray et al., 2004). Spiritual needs are characterized "by normal expressions of a person's inner being that motivates (sic) the search for meaning in all experiences" and as "a dynamic relationship with others, self and whatever the person values" (Narayanasamy, 2007, p. 35). The dying process is partially shaped by how one responds to the spiritual challenges and subsequent needs that emerge (Miller et al., 2005). The process of meeting one's spiritual needs involves spiritual seeking and spiritual struggle (Peteet & Balboni, 2013). So, for example, one may have a spiritual need to forgive a family member, which requires a series of steps to take responsibility for such reconciliation. For people who are religious, spiritual needs might be associated with religious needs (Glasper, 2011). Examples include the need to pray, discuss religious beliefs, or engage in religious rites (Nixon & Narayanasamy, 2010). When spirituality is important to hospice patients, hospice social workers need the capacity to identify spiritual needs and help patients address them (Kellehear, 2000; Langegard & Ahlberg, 2009; Peteet & Balboni, 2013).

TYPES OF SPIRITUAL NEEDS

Authors across disciplines have identified diverse spiritual needs associated with the dying process. The meeting of spiritual needs in preparation for death is what Byock (1996) calls "task-work" (p. 247). Hospice patients have to be willing to engage in this task-work, but the meeting of spiritual needs has the potential to facilitate a sense of completion, satisfaction, and even mastery in life (Byock, 1996; Edwards et al., 2010). Hospice social workers can help by understanding the most common spiritual needs of patients with terminal illness (see table 3.1). As seen in table 3.1, information about

TABLE 3.1   Common Spiritual Needs and Means of Coping in Patients with Terminal Illness

Involvement and control	Obtain information that enables one to exercise control over one's life, actively prepare for death, experience self-reliance and independence, have input into one's own life, have information about one's own care, stay as independent as possible, have things in life stay the same, have information about family and friends, be helped by others, feel useful, maintain sense of self-worth, retain an active role with family and friends, talk about death and dying.
Religious activities	Pray, read/use phrases from a religious text/literature, attend religious services, seek comfort and support from church, talk with someone about religious issues, be with people who share religious beliefs, visit with clergy/chaplain, *seek religious reconciliation, experience divine forgiveness and support, practice religious rites/sacraments, engage in discussions about God.**
Spiritual activities	Read/use inspirational material, sing/listen to music, meditate, have quiet time, indulge in spiritual self-care, talk with someone about spiritual issues/meaning of life/peace of mind, be with people who share spiritual beliefs.
Finish business	Review one's life, evaluate life accomplishments, finish life tasks, come to terms with present situation, resolve bitter feelings, overcome fears, find meaning, gain closure, receive and offer forgiveness, accept pending death, *process grief, seek peace and reconciliation, reunite with others.**
Positive outlook	Think happy thoughts, maintain an open mind, laugh, appreciate the significance of the moment, take one day at a time, be around children, talk about day-to-day things, see others smiling, feel hope/trust/affirmation/sense of purpose.
Companionship	Be with family, be with friends, talk with others, talk about day-to-day things, help care for others, give and receive love, feel connected to social world, *experience a sense of mutuality.**
Experience nature	Look outside, be outside, have flowers in the room, garden, have pets.

* Spiritual needs in italics were not reported by patients but are included here to lend insight into other potential spiritual needs based on a comprehensive review of palliative- and hospice-care research.

Sources: Balboni et al., 2007; Edwards et al., 2010; Hermann, 2001, 2006, 2007; Kellehear, 2000; Moadel et al., 1999; Murray et al., 2004, 2007; Tan, Braunack-Mayer, & Beilby, 2005.

spiritual needs lends insight into means of coping. Spiritual needs in italics were not reported by patients but were included to lend insight into other potential spiritual needs based on a review of palliative- and hospice-care research. Spiritual needs are also likely to be relative to multiple factors, a point addressed later in this chapter. For now, three studies that delineate the spiritual needs of patients will be reviewed. Edwards et al. (2010) conducted a systematic review of research that included patient reports and observations of informal caregivers and health-care providers to identify a patient's spiritual needs. Hermann (2001) conducted a qualitative study with hospice patients for a more in-depth discussion of spiritual needs. A follow-up study by Hermann (2006) developed an instrument to measure levels of spiritual need. Each study takes a different approach in describing the spiritual needs of patients. Even though this is not a systematic review of the literature, it does focus on available research that specifically asks patients to describe their own spiritual needs.

A Systematic Review of Qualitative Studies

Edwards et al. (2010) systematically analyzed qualitative studies published between 2001 and 2009 on spirituality and palliative care. They found 19 studies, of which 11 had interviewed patients. Five studies specifically examined what patients reported as being their spiritual needs. These studies suggested that patients needed the opportunity to finish business, experience involvement and control, and have a positive outlook. To finish business, patients might engage in life review through reminiscing and seeking to understand life as it unfolded. This process might further involve reconciliation for a new closeness with others. Patients may process grief and, eventually, acceptance of pending death. The second spiritual need was the need for involvement and control. Patients wanted information that enabled them to exercise control over their lives and remain involved in family life. This included the need to actively prepare for death. The exercise of self-control further included the desire to be self-reliant and independent. The third spiritual need was for a positive outlook. A positive outlook was described as embracing happy thoughts, maintaining an open mind, sharing humor and laughter, seeing smiles on the faces of others, and appreciating the significance of the moment. When the authors reviewed collective responses from patients, informal caregivers, and health-care providers, Edwards et al. found more evidence to suggest that patients needed forgiveness and reconciliation, ability to let go and accept their circumstances, and opportunity for life review and reminiscence. They also found patients needed social engagement that involved talking about death and dying as well as to talk about ordinary things for a sense of normality.

Six Categories of Spiritual Needs

Although the study by Hermann (2001) was included in the review by Edwards et al. (2010), Hermann's work provides a broader range of spiritual needs and more detailed account of each based on interviews with patients. Hermann interviewed 19 hospice patients and identified 29 spiritual needs. Hermann found that most of these patients associated spiritual needs with religious needs, but patients also described many other spiritual needs as well. The author suggested that the spiritual needs identified were related, in that they helped inform life purpose and meaning. Hence, there was some overlap between spiritual needs, and some appeared to be related to biopsychosocial needs. The author identified six themes under which spiritual needs were organized as seen in figure 3.1. These themes included need for religion, need for companionship, need for involvement and control, need to finish business, need to experience nature, and need for a positive outlook. Each need is summarized in the following sections.

NEED FOR RELIGION

The first spiritual need identified was for religion. This need was said to include the need to pray and rely on inspirational materials, such as religious scripture, for strength. The need to attend church services was identified as being important, but participation was limited, given the fragile health of patients. This need was further expressed by listening to a recording of the church service, reading about church news, visiting with one's religious leader, and singing and/or listening to religious songs.

NEED FOR COMPANIONSHIP

Every patient reported the need for companionship as a primary need. Patients said they simply needed to be with others. Others were needed to provide support, which may have included just spending time with others and talking with them about everyday things. About half of the patients

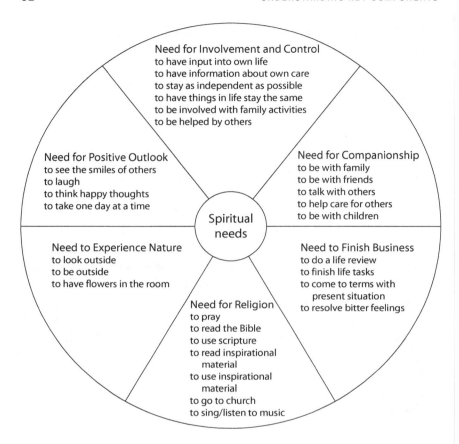

FIGURE 3.1 Thematic organization of spiritual needs.
Source: Hermann (2001).

said they had a desire to help others, for example, through praying for them. Several patients reported a desire to be around children, as this reminded them of the continuity of life.

NEED FOR INVOLVEMENT AND CONTROL

The need for involvement and control was said to be significant as it related to other spiritual needs. Hermann said this category was necessary to reflect the distinct need for patients to be involved in decision making. This required access to information, for example, to make health-care decisions and resolve family issues. This extended into the need to maintain one's independence as part of self-care. Involvement further enabled care for others by, for example, being present for family meals.

NEED TO FINISH BUSINESS

The need to finish business involved reflecting on life experiences to understand why things happened the way they did and how these experiences helped shaped these patients as people. The need to finish business also related to living life more fully, resolving issues such as legal and financial matters, or fulfilling aspirations, for example, plans to travel. Finishing business therefore involved reconciling both past and present concerns. Beyond celebrating joys, this need to finish business may require the resolution of anger to experience peace at the end of life.

NEED TO EXPERIENCE NATURE

Although less frequent, there were patients who expressed a need to interact with nature to experience spirituality. This involved having the need to take a walk outside and/or to look at the grass and trees from inside or from the back porch. One example referenced in the study was related to an appreciation for cut flowers from the patient's own garden; however, it was unclear whether this example was more of a reminder of that patient's life before terminal illness rather than of the spiritual need to experience nature.

NEED FOR POSITIVE OUTLOOK

Several patients expressed a need to maintain a positive outlook that was supported by cheerful people who smiled and shared funny stories. Hermann related several examples of patients who described their efforts to cultivate a focus on faith and hope in God through meditation on inspirational materials. Several respondents reported the need to focus on living one day at a time. Hermann may have included this example to illustrate how focusing on the present provided a means of distraction and implied the need to believe it was possible to make it though.

A Measure for Levels of Spiritual Need

Hermann (2006) later used these findings to create an instrument to measure levels of spiritual need. The instrument was evaluated by other researchers and completed by 100 hospice patients to determine the accuracy of indicators for spiritual needs. This process included asking whether patients experienced these needs and whether they believed these needs were spiritual in nature. During various stages of analysis, 10 items were deleted, and a remaining 17 items were divided into five subscales somewhat differently than in Hermann (2001) to address measurement issues. The final subscales and items included the spiritual need for (1) religion, as indicated by the need to pray and go to religious services; (2) community, as indicated by the need to be with family and friends and have information about family and friends; (3) inspiration, as indicated by the need to sing/listen to music, read a religious text, talk with someone about religious or spiritual issues, and be with people who share one's religious beliefs; (4) spiritual activities, as indicated by the need to read inspirational material, use inspirational material, and use phrases from a religious text; and (5) a positive outlook, as indicated by the need to laugh, be around children, think happy thoughts, talk about day-to-day things, and see others smiling. Even though the need to finish business was deleted in this analysis, the author suggested that it may still be important given support found in the literature. Hermann's evidence of common spiritual needs as well as spiritual needs that are unique to each patient (2001, 2006) leads to questions about what factors contribute to the experience of spiritual needs and risk for unmet spiritual needs.

DIVERSITY ISSUES AND RISK FOR UNMET SPIRITUAL NEEDS

The dying process, like every life transition, is marked by developmental challenges. These developmental challenges can threaten personhood, as physical decline entails loss. Although the focus of this chapter has been on identifying common spiritual needs, there are biopsychosocial needs that also have the potential to shape a patient's spiritual experience. As described in chapter 2, the experience of spirituality and its related spiritual needs and resources can vary from one patient to the next. In fact, research suggests that spiritual needs vary according to patient demographics, treatment setting, and other circumstances (Barber, 2012). Therefore, spiritual needs are not isolated or static factors but must be considered in relation to other biopsychosocial factors that can change over time (Kellehear, 2000). This makes understanding patients' spiritual needs a challenge for both patients and hospice social workers. Awareness of spiritual needs requires a level of insight that one may not or does not want to have. A patient may not feel comfortable discussing spiritual needs with a hospice social worker for fear of judgment (Sheldon, 2000). A hospice social worker may not see a patient's spiritual needs if they are obscured, for example, by physical needs for medical care (Grant et al., 2004). Therefore, just as patients' biopsychosocial needs change over time, their spiritual needs may also change. This necessitates continued efforts for hospice social workers to engage in assessment and intervention that is congruent with a patient's expectations, resources, and capacity to benefit from care (Murray et al., 2004; Wynne, 2013).

One of the challenges is that most research on spiritual needs is based on the experience of elderly, white, and Judeo-Christian patients with cancer, so more research is needed to determine potential variation across hospice patients (Draper, 2011; Edwards et al., 2010; Hermann, 2001, 2006; Peteet & Balboni, 2013). A number of studies have suggested that the experience and expression of spiritual needs can vary based on a range of factors such as race (Balboni et al., 2007; Branch, Torke, Brown-Haithco, 2006; Bullock, 2011; Johnson, Elbert-Avila, & Tulsky, 2005; Raghavan, Smith, & Arnold, 2010), gender (Chochinov & Cann, 2005; Hermann, 2007), age (Barber, 2012; Buck, Overcash, & McMillan, 2009; Moberg, 2005; Peteet & Balboni, 2013; Walter, 2002), culture (Ando et al., 2009; Balboni et al., 2007; Bullock, 2011; Chochinov & Cann, 2005; Draper, 2011), marital status (Chochinov & Cann, 2005; Emanuel, Alpert, Baldwin, & Emanuel, 2000), religious affiliation (Gay, Lynxwiler, & Peek, 2001; Glasper, 2011), religious/spiritual commitment (Balboni et al., 2007; Okon, 2005; Peteet & Balboni, 2013), health condition (type of illness; Chochinov & Cann, 2005; Grant et al., 2004; Murray et al, 2004; Murray, Kendall, Grant, Boyd, Barclay, & Sheikh, 2007; Nixon & Narayanasamy, 2010), trajectory of illness (change in medical status, types of symptoms, functional capacity, and duration; Balboni et al., 2007; Grant et al., 2004; Hermann, 2007; Murray et al., 2004, 2007; Nixon & Narayanasamy, 2010; Okon, 2005), and treatment setting/community resources (Balboni et al., 2007; Chochinov & Cann, 2005; Dzul-Church, Cimino, Adler, Wong, & Anderson, 2010; Hermann, 2007). A full review is beyond the scope of this chapter, but several studies will be discussed to demonstrate how a combination of factors may shape spiritual needs and subsequent risk for spiritual needs to go unmet.

Type of Illness and Illness Trajectory

Murray et al. (2004) conducted a longitudinal study in the United Kingdom with patients and their informal caregivers to determine whether there were different spiritual needs relative to type of illness and illness trajectory. The authors conducted 149 in-depth interviews every 3 months for up to 1 year with 20 patients with end-stage heart failure and 20 patients with inoperable lung cancer and their informal caregivers. This allowed data to be collected at different points during the progression of illness. The authors indicated that patients reported the need for meaning and forgiveness, to give and receive love, to feel connected to their social world, to feel useful, to maintain a sense of self-worth, and to retain an active role with family and friends. For those who were religious, there was a need to seek comfort and support from their churches and a need for prayer. Patients reported individual strategies for spiritual self-care, for example, through activities that provided a distraction. Murray et al. found that patients often resisted expressing their spiritual needs to avoid upsetting others. There were some changes in spiritual needs and experience of spiritual distress that were specific to type of illness and illness trajectory.

The authors observed that patients with heart failure struggled to find meaning in life given the chronic nature of the disease. Patients also experienced episodes of acute deterioration. Patients said they felt abandoned, hopeless, and isolated. Increased disability and need for assistance was experienced as depersonalizing and degrading, which led to an altered self-image. Death was sudden, so patients were unable to plan for it. For patients with lung cancer, there was a more defined progression from diagnosis to end of life. It was observed that each phase led to new spiritual challenges, although the authors did not describe the experiences in terms of spiritual needs, but instead focused on signs of spiritual distress. This might suggest the authors considered spiritual needs and spiritual distress as being related. The authors summarized by saying that lung cancer patients experienced despair upon first diagnosis that involved questions about why they were sick and what to expect. Patients felt a sense of loss of control offset by periods of increased sense of purpose as they focused on defeating the disease during the treatment phase. Patients experienced renewed hope when they felt better. When symptoms returned, patients experienced doubt marked by more questions about their faith and self-blame. Therefore, over the course of their illness, patients with lung cancer struggled with existential questions that entailed feelings of doubt and fear followed by a renewed sense of purpose and hope.

Murray et al. (2007) followed up by combining the data of Murray et al. (2004) with data from a similar study by Grant et al. (2004) conducted in Ireland. The purpose of this study was to examine whether a patient's spiritual needs presented in combination with psychosocial needs relative to type of illness and illness trajectory. The authors explored the experience of 24 patients with end-stage heart failure and 24 patients with inoperable lung cancer. To determine spiritual needs, the authors asked patients to describe how they were doing spiritually. Spiritual needs were associated with spiritual distress, and the opposite of spiritual distress was identified as spiritual well-being. Spiritual distress and spiritual well-being were not further defined by the authors. The authors compared patient responses to see whether spiritual needs emerged at specific times during the course of illness.

For patients with heart failure, spiritual needs varied throughout their illness. Spiritual distress increased as patients questioned their value and place in the world and experienced a loss of identity and growing dependence. The authors noted that illness and suffering also led to positive feelings such as hope, trust, love, and forgiveness. Some patients said they felt affirmed by their doctor. There were patients who were comforted by their religious beliefs; however, there were also patients who feared divine judgment or indifference. As death approached, patients asked more explicit questions about, for example, what might happen after death. For patients with lung cancer, spiritual needs and risk for spiritual distress more clearly occurred at specific times and were closely associated with psychological distress. The times when spiritual needs were most evident was at the time of diagnosis, at the time of recurrence of symptoms, during the terminal stage, and at the end of treatment. At diagnosis, patients searched for answers to explain why they had to experience suffering and confront pending death. Patients who returned home at the end of treatment struggled to retain a sense of self-worth and value to others as part of normal life. As the disease progressed and symptoms recurred, some patients evaluated life accomplishments and what they needed to gain closure and struggled to gain a sense of purpose. The terminal phase leading up to the end of treatment involved acceptance of pending death. Some people worried about the afterlife, but others expressed confidence in the continuation of a spiritual life after death. Murray et al. (2007) acknowledged that these results may not reflect the experience of all patients, particularly those from different backgrounds or circumstances not captured in the study.

Gender, Education Level, Illness Trajectory, and Treatment Setting

Hermann (2007) surveyed 100 hospice patients to determine the degree to which their spiritual needs had been met. Each patient completed the Spiritual Needs Inventory (Hermann, 2001, 2006). Hermann also asked patients to rate their life satisfaction. Overall, spirituality seemed to be very important to these patients, and their spiritual needs were met at a moderate to high rate as they neared the end of life. The need to pray was rated as having the greatest importance, followed by the need to think happy thoughts, laugh, and see people smiling. Spiritual needs that could be met independently and that were not dependent on functional status were said to be met at a higher rate. The need to pray was the most common need that was met by 96 percent of patients. The need to sing or listen to music, talk about day-to-day things, use inspirational materials, use phrases from a religious text, and see the smiles of others was perceived as being met by 80–89 percent of patients. The need to have information about family and friends, talk with someone about spiritual issues, think happy thoughts, be around children, and be with people who share one's spiritual beliefs was perceived as met by 70–79 percent of the patients. The need to read religious texts, read inspirational materials, laugh, and be with family and friends was perceived as met by 60–68 percent of the patients. The need to go to religious services was met by 30 percent of the patients.

Although unmet spiritual needs were reported at a lower rate, these unmet spiritual needs seemed to be relative to several factors. Patients who reported having more unmet spiritual needs were women, patients living in a nursing home or inpatient hospice unit, and patients with lower levels of education. The authors suggested that women were at higher risk for unmet spiritual needs given the potential for women in general to have more spiritual needs (or to at least express them and seek help to meet them) than men. They proposed that the spiritual needs patients could meet on their own were met at a higher rate than spiritual needs that required the assistance of others. Most patients reported that the spiritual need to go to religious services and other spiritual needs that involved being with others were often unmet. Perhaps patients receiving hospice care in a nursing home or inpatient unit had poorer functional status or fewer social supports, which reduced their ability to meet their own needs or access spiritual resources. This seems to suggest that hospice-care providers in these facilities failed to provide patients with adequate spiritual care. The same would be true for patients with lower levels of education who might have needed more assistance in identifying ways to get their spiritual needs met. Again, homogeneity in the study's sample made it impossible to determine whether spiritual needs were relative to symptoms of terminal illness or cultural factors, so the results may not reflect the experience of patients from different backgrounds or circumstances.

Race, Culture, Religiosity, Illness Trajectory, and Community Resources

One study provides insight into the risk for unmet spiritual needs in a more diverse population with cancer based on race and ethnicity (Balboni et al., 2007). Balboni et al. surveyed 230 patients living in the south and northeast United States with advanced cancer, of whom 61 percent were white and 39 percent were nonwhite. The authors found that 88 percent considered religion to be at least somewhat important. Religion was reported as being important to 89 percent of African Americans and 79 percent of Hispanics compared with 59 percent of white patients. Spiritual needs were only minimally met by the medical system in 72 percent of the patients and by a religious community in 47 percent of the patients. Spiritual needs were not met by either the medical system or by a religious community in 42 percent of the patients. Greater spiritual support from outside and within the medical system was significantly associated with patient quality of life. Among religious patients, 52 percent of African Americans said they were completely supported by religious communities more frequently compared with 26 percent of Hispanics and 19 percent of white patients. Fifty-two percent of patients received visits from chaplains or clergy. These visits were said to have provided at least some comfort in 100 percent of Hispanics, 94 percent of African Americans, and 83 percent of white patients, but 3 percent of the patients reported that these visits made them uncomfortable. Degree of religiosity did not vary based on age. Fifty-six percent of the patients reported attending religious services at least once a month, but this decreased to 44 percent after diagnosis. Conversely, 47 percent of the patients reported engaging in private spiritual activities at least daily, which increased to 61 percent after diagnosis. Degree of religiosity was also significantly associated with a desire for life-extending measures.

Taken together, these results suggest that a range of factors are related to spiritual needs. The experience of unmet spiritual needs is particularly disturbing because patients should have access to spiritual support throughout the provision of hospice care. This support may be more important for patients who are religious and/or report having more spiritual needs, such as patients who are female, African American, and/or Hispanic. The ability of patients to meet their own spiritual needs may change along an illness's trajectory, ranging from the point of diagnosis to when the symptoms of illness increase. Limited spiritual support through the medical system may be compounded by limited spiritual support in the community. For example, Dzul-Church et al. (2010) found that it was common for patients with a history of difficult life experience such as substance abuse, mental health issues, homelessness, and imprisonment to have more limited resources that profoundly shaped their experience of terminal illness. The authors noted that these patients had estrangement in life but did not want similar isolation in death. This was believed to influence patient reliance on health-care providers as "family"; however, patients said it seemed providers felt rushed and failed to listen to them or to provide desired help in making plans for death. Some patients wanted to reconcile relationships, but they were not provided assistance and lacked the resources to gain closure. Patients wanted health-care providers to affirm them as "unique, complex person[s] in the context of their histories and values" (p. 699). Spirituality played an important role in self-care, but patients said they also needed better relationships with providers, access to chaplaincy services, and home-based services for support.

CONCLUSION

Research suggests that there are common spiritual needs as well as unique spiritual needs that are shaped by a range of biopsychosocial factors (Allamani, 2007). The meeting of spiritual needs is essential in end-of-life care (Langegard & Ahlberg, 2009), as it supports patients who seek wholeness in the midst of profound vulnerability (Goldberg & Crespo, 2003). Advances in medicine may extend the time patients have to transform spiritual challenges into the experience of enhanced life meaning and purpose (Grant, 2007). Hospice social workers can support patients in this process. As described by the Hospice Foundation of America (2005):

> Once the needs of dying persons are understood and accepted, we are then able to refocus the goals of care. Instead of hoping for a cure, the dying person has a right to hope for a comfortable death, free of pain and discomfort. The dying person can retain the hope of finding or re-finding the value of his or her life; of resolving what was previously not able to be resolved; discovering or re-discovering spirituality. The dying person may renew a quest for answers to great existential questions. It is not unusual for the dying person to find deep reservoirs of faith that were never suspected before. There is much that a dying person can hope for.
>
> (p. 8)

Most importantly, hospice patients have needs they themselves consider spiritual in nature. Research in this area further suggests that these spiritual needs can be met. The type of spiritual need provides direction for how this might be done. For example, a spiritual need for involvement and control might be met through helping patients stay as independent as possible. Some spiritual needs may not be met due to a patient's health condition (Hermann, 2006). This could reveal other biopsychosocial needs. Spiritual needs are complex and so is the process of addressing them. Chapter 4 explores potential consequences of unmet needs and resources for patients to build and/or sustain spiritual resilience.

4

Spiritual Suffering

SPIRITUALITY CAN HAVE A PROFOUND effect on how patients cope with terminal illness (Hills et al., 2005; Lukoff, n.d.). Spirituality can be a source of relief or related to significant distress (Edwards et al., 2010; Murray et al., 2004; Pargament, Feuille, & Burdzy, 2011; Peteet & Balboni, 2013; Puchalski, 2008a). Spiritual needs to understand "Why me?" and "What happens next?" can prompt spiritual distress when there are no answers (Hospice and Palliative Nurses Association [HPNA], 2013). Spiritual resources can help patients meet spiritual needs as they face the end of life. Therefore, terminal illness can evoke a range of thoughts, feelings, and behaviors that have implications for life quality (NHPCO, 2007). If patient functioning is compromised in the process, then hospice social workers should be able to help in coordination with interdisciplinary team members (Hills et al., 2005). This chapter begins by exploring the experience of spiritual suffering and how spiritual suffering might influence biopsychosocial and spiritual functioning that ends with a call for help.

DEFINING SPIRITUAL SUFFERING

Some variation of the term "spiritual suffering" has been used across disciplines. Spiritual suffering has been identified as the experience of despair, spiritual pain, spiritual distress, spiritual struggles, spiritual problems, spiritual concerns, spiritual issues, existential pain, existential distress, existential suffering, existential concerns, religious pain, religious distress, and religious struggles (Chochinov & Cann, 2005; Exline, Prince-Paul,

Root, & Peereboom, 2013; Heyse-Moore, 1996; Mako, Galek, & Poppito, 2006; Pargament, 2007; University of Alabama, n.d.). Cicely Saunders, the founder of the hospice movement, believed that spiritual pain was part of the "total pain" experienced by patients requiring "total care" (Saunders, 2005, p. 34; Heyse-Moore, 1996). In a study to measure the experience of spiritual pain in patients with terminal illness, Mako et al. (2006) simply described spiritual pain as "a pain deep in your being that is not physical" (p. 1108). Spiritual pain can lead one to feel disconnected or experience a loss of self or an internal void (Chaturvedi, 2007; Elias, Giglio, & Pimenta, 2008). There are likely to be questions about one's belief or value system that once inspired hope, strength, and life meaning (Nixon & Narayanasamy, 2010; Wintz & Cooper, 2003). Millison (1988) said it is this failure to find meaning that results in spiritual pain, while Narayanasamy (2007) suggests spiritual pain is caused by disharmony in mind, body, and spirit. NANDA established spiritual distress as a nursing diagnosis in 1978. Spiritual distress is an "impaired ability to experience and integrate meaning and purpose in life through a person's connectedness with self, others, art, music, literature, nature, or a power greater than oneself" (Puchalski et al., 2006, p. 405; Lukoff, n.d.; Puchalski, 2008b). Likewise, other authors have suggested that existential pain results when life experiences do not measure up to one's expectations and fail to make life meaningful (Chochinov & Cann, 2005; Edwards et al., 2010; Walter, 2002). No matter which name or cause is applied, spiritual suffering is real and can have serious implications (NHPCO, 2007).

Pain Versus Suffering

Pain and suffering may seem like one in the same, but Goldberg and Crespo (2003) suggest that they are different. Pain becomes suffering when it seems to diminish one's humanity or that which sustains personhood (Cassell, 1982). Suffering is also socially constructed and shared with others who further define pain as suffering. For example, childbirth is more traditionally associated with the experience of pain. Although the pain of labor can be severe, it is not typically associated with suffering, because pain is considered a normal part of birth, necessary to produce a child. Cassell (1982) suggests that pain may be equated with suffering when a person feels "out of control, when the pain is overwhelming, when the source of the pain is unknown, when the meaning of the pain is dire, or when the pain is chronic" (p. 641). In the case of childbirth, pain is time limited under controlled conditions. This makes the pain more bearable and thus less likely to be viewed as suffering. The outcome is a child who adds new meaning to life, which makes the pain all the more bearable. It is a natural part of life to experience birth as well as death. However, unlike birth, death presents the potential for a unique experience of suffering (Byock, 1996).

The Dying Process: A Universal, Unique Experience

Terminal illness may include the experience of physical suffering, but it can also evoke psychological, social, and spiritual suffering. Yang, Staps, and Hijmans (2010) analyzed the experiences of 15 patients in the Netherlands to discover how they coped with the dying process. They found that spiritual suffering described as being prompted by an existential crisis involved a dynamic process of self-transformation. The authors found that patients needed to have some sense of purpose that directed activity and enabled a sense of control over life. Pending death threatened this process of meaning making. Patients initially tried to approach terminal illness as though it could be cured. Over time, perspectives changed and became more present oriented to enable patients to manage daily challenges. This reduced the stress and anxiety associated with facing an unknown future. When physical deterioration made pending death unavoidable, a perceived loss of control and crisis occurred that resulted in the experience of mourning. When patients allowed themselves to process grief, a new sense of meaning emerged. For some, this meant a new sense of connection with larger humanity, particularly with other patients going through the dying process. This helped patients feel less fearful of death. It took additional time for patients to internalize this new understanding and operate within it.

Yang et al. (2010) said most of the patients had the courage to engage in the process of constructing, internalizing, and then operating within this new reality. This process required patients to manage intense emotions of living within a meaningless void before they could come to accept the inevitability of death. In the process of reconstructing the meaning of their lives, patients rediscovered themselves, including their histories, identities, and characters. This process was said to enrich patients' lives and enhanced their ability to love others. The authors suggested that this process also seemed to help patients experience a more authentic self. For example, there were some patients who focused intensely on being in touch with the present moment. Patients prioritized activities, which seemed to enhance self-esteem and depth of experience. In accepting death, patients were able to redirect their limited energy to meeting their daily needs. There were some patients who felt they were part of a greater whole. This "meant a deep connectedness with mankind, nature, or with a transcendental dimension like infinity or God . . . [or] with themselves" (p. 61). Although, connectedness was difficult for patients to describe, it seemed to entail a decrease in loneliness. It inspired trust, which offset feelings of powerlessness and panic. Most importantly, it could not be forced: "This experiential dimension of meaning cannot be evoked consciously or at will. Apart from genuinely going through a process of mourning, it often also seems to be important to seek a quiet situation, a walk through the woods or meditation, wherein such an experience of meaning may be 'received'" (p. 61).

The process of coping with existential crisis, which entailed finding new meaning in life, was described as a lived experience of spirituality. The manner in which this process unfolded could not be forced, but rather it was perhaps a natural product of working through a range of emotions associated with accepting pending death. How a patient responded to existential crisis seemed to profoundly shape the spiritual quality of the experience. Overall, this process included (1) feelings of loss that led to a process of mourning, (2) receptivity to a new understanding of pending death, and (3) attribution of meaning and experience of meaning associated with pending death. The authors noted that they were surprised by observations that suggested there were many different moments during the course of illness in which existential crisis manifested. It was observed that an existential crisis emerged even when death was no longer a threat. During this coping process, patients reported intense feelings of loneliness. They were ambivalent about sharing their experiences; while sharing made them feel vulnerable, they expressed the need to talk more about their experiences. Therefore, even though one aspect of suffering was the need to find meaning in the experience of dying, it also seemed important to have someone to share this with. Religion was not described as a central component of this process, which could be due to this study being conducted in the Netherlands, a more secular society than the United States.

Those with terminal illness have different personalities and life experiences. What is valued and defines personhood has implications for the meaning attached to one's experience of terminal illness. Suffering may be in response to changes in one's physical body, a loss of professional status, the new social role as patient, dependence on family members, questions about eternal life, and many other things. If these changes are perceived as losses, the types of losses and how one interprets the impact of these losses are a part of what makes the dying process unique. As described by Cassell (1982):

> Suffering is ultimately a personal matter. Patients sometimes report suffering when one does not expect it, or do not report suffering when one does expect it. Furthermore, a person can suffer enormously at the distress of another, especially a loved one. In some theologies, suffering has been seen as bringing one closer to God. This "function" of suffering is at once its glorification and its relief. If, through great pain or deprivation, someone is brought closer to a cherished goal, that person may have no sense of having suffered but may instead feel enormous triumph. To an observer, however, only the deprivation may be apparent.
>
> (pp. 640–641)

As a result, the meaning associated with the experience of dying is personal and individual, but it is also shared with humanity and others in similar circumstances. Suffering may be considered a threat to some, whereas for others it may enable the expression of one's authentic self, a deeper connection with others, and a new sense of life meaning (Langegard & Ahlberg, 2009). Spirituality may be an important aspect of the dying process, a fact that requires hospice social workers to be able to identify potential signs of spiritual suffering (Yang et al., 2010), particularly when other forms of suffering are more visible or concrete and time is of the essence (Exline et al., 2013).

A HOLISTIC CONNECTION

There are different ways to experience spiritual suffering, and this influences how spiritual suffering may manifest (HPNA, 2013; Narayanasamy, 2007). Most authors describe spiritual suffering as being evidenced by biological, psychological, social, and spiritual symptoms (Büssing, Balzat, & Heusser, 2010; Byock, 1996; Chochinov & Cann, 2005; Cornette, 2005; Elias et al., 2008; Exline et al., 2013; Heyse-Moore, 1996; Lukoff, n.d.; Mako et al., 2006; Murray et al., 2004; Narayanasamy, 2007; NHPCO, 2007; Nixon & Narayanasamy, 2010; Puchalski, 2008a, 2013; University of Alabama, n.d.; Wintz & Cooper, 2003). Overlap in signs of spiritual suffering can make the experience more difficult to recognize and address for both patients and hospice social workers (Puchalski, 2013). More research is needed to clarify the exact nature of spiritual suffering, but it helps to start with how patients have described their own experiences.

In a study by Mako et al. (2006), chaplains interviewed 57 patients hospitalized with an advanced stage cancer about spiritual suffering, measured as spiritual pain. The patients were asked to describe spiritual pain as well as the frequency and intensity. Patients were provided with a preliminary definition of spiritual pain as being "a pain deep in your being that is not physical" (p. 1108). The authors found that more than 96 percent of the patients reported experiencing some spiritual pain. For some patients, spiritual pain was described more or less in physical terms, as seen in the following example:

> One patient observed that his spiritual pain feels like "everything is breaking down and I'm not here anymore." This sense of existential annihilation is a powerful realization that one is separating from life as one ebbs toward death. For others, the sense of spiritual pain is inextricably linked with the physical. For instance, one person indicated that he could not tell the difference between physical and spiritual pain. Other patients described their spiritual pain in bodily terms, "like all the elements of my body are diminishing," "a big lump in my stomach," and "an ache all over my body." Another patient observed that his spiritual pain "feels like a bullet hit my heart."
>
> (p. 1110)

Mako et al. further observed that more than half the patients manifested emotions and used emotional terms to express their spiritual pain. Patients used words such as "regret," "anxiety," and "despair." The authors proposed that patients used this approach because it gave them the words to describe the intangible aspects of spirituality. Therefore, it was unclear whether patients were able to fully articulate their experience of spiritual pain.

This study does suggest that the way patients interpret and express spiritual pain could have implications for how they experience and cope with spiritual pain (Elias et al., 2008).

Based on the meta-analysis of qualitative palliative-care research by Edwards et al. (2010), patients reported multiple signs of spiritual suffering that the authors described as spiritual distress. The authors observed that spiritual distress was "mixed with and impinged on physical, psychological, social and financial distress" (p. 760). These signs were presented all together, but are divided under what seemed to be associated dimensions in table 4.1 for clarification. These results were found to be largely congruent with other literature. Signs of spiritual distress (in italics in the table) were not reported by patients in this study but are included to lend insight into other potential signs of spiritual suffering and are based on a review of palliative- and hospice-care research (see table 4.1). Psychosocial symptoms were identified most often as signs of spiritual distress. Edwards et al. found that the feeling of fear, especially the fear of death, was the most significant emotion. This translated into feeling insecure, nervous, and overwhelmed, especially at night. This anxiety was further related to physical symptoms such as panic attacks or insomnia. The authors noted other negative feelings, but those seemed to be indicative of spiritual/existential symptoms such as hopelessness, lack of meaning or purpose, and despair. In fact, the authors noted that the literature suggested that it was difficult to determine whether a patient was experiencing spiritual distress or clinical depression. Patients also reported symptoms akin to social death (Callahan, 2011a). Loss of physical abilities led to a greater dependence on others and feelings of uselessness. Patients felt unable to engage in traditional family and social roles. Some patients felt rejected and abandoned by others.

Types of Spiritual Suffering

The work of Pargament (2007) and associates (Ellison & Lee, 2010; Pargament, Murray-Swank, Magyar, & Ano, 2005) describes spiritual suffering as being associated with interpersonal, intrapersonal, and/or divine struggles. This model employs a religious worldview; however, even if a patient does not report a religious affiliation, similar spiritual struggles might apply given past affiliation or experiences. Interpersonal spiritual struggles involve having problems with families, friends, and other groups. Patients may feel

TABLE 4.1 Biopsychosocial-Spiritual Signs of Spiritual Suffering

BIOLOGICAL	PSYCHOLOGICAL	SOCIAL	SPIRITUAL[†]
Panic attacks, insomnia, restlessness, decreased physical abilities, physical discomfort, worsening physical symptoms, *intractable pain, crying, treatment noncompliance*[*]	Fear (of the unknown, of death), insecurity, nervousness, anxiety, feeling overwhelmed, hopelessness, helplessness, resignation, emptiness, depression, anger, cynicism, bitterness, impatience, irritability, frustration, feelings of being victimized, guilt/shame (related to self), *uncertainty, anguish, loneliness, confusion, grief, annihilation, psychosis*[*]	Blaming others for condition; taking pain out on others for release; loss of self (in relation to others); altered body image; loss in relationships; forced dependency; low self-worth; feelings of uselessness; loss of family and social roles; assuming the "invalid" role; feelings of being abandoned, rejected, and/or neglected by others; guilt/shame (related to others); *alienation; clinging; withdrawal; isolation; inability to forgive; resentment*[*]	Guilt (related to God); feelings of being punished, judged, abandoned, rejected, and/or neglected by God; loss of meaning/faith (questions such as "Why me?"); despair; *disagreements with clergy, members of faith community, family members or friends; demoralization; power of negative spiritual or demonic forces*[*]

[*] Signs of spiritual suffering in italics were not reported by patients but are included here to lend insight into other potential signs of spiritual suffering based on a review of palliative- and hospice-care research.

[†] Includes religious and existential concerns.

Sources: Byock, 1996; Carroll, 2001; Chochinov & Cann, 2005; Cornette, 2005; Edwards et al., 2010; Ellison & Lee, 2010; Heyse-Moore, 1996; Hills et al., 2005; HPNA, 2013; Lukoff, n.d.; Mako et al., 2006; Murray et al., 2004; Narayanasamy, 2007; Nixon & Narayanasamy, 2010; NHPCO, 2007; Pargament, 2007; Pargament et al., 2005; Puchalski, 2008a 2013; Wintz & Cooper, 2003; Yang et al., 2010.

abandoned by their church or alienated when they see members engage in behaviors that contradict their religious beliefs. They might disagree with religious leaders or church doctrine. Spiritual struggles may further undermine the spiritual bond between family members. Patients may not agree with family members or friends about spiritual or religious matters. They may question whose side God is on or seek God's punishment for those who hurt them. The second type of spiritual struggle is intrapersonal. Intrapersonal spiritual struggle can manifest as doubts about spiritual values or religious beliefs. This may involve difficulty in maintaining behavior that is congruent with one's ideals. Patients may question why they are alive. They may struggle with guilt for having doubts or for failing to live up to their own expectations. Tension between the individual and the divine represents the third form of spiritual struggle. This might involve having more specific questions about the nature of one's relationship with God. Patients might feel punished by God, angry with God, or abandoned by God. Patients may fear they let God down and question God's love for them. Struggles with the divine could further include a belief in the power of negative spiritual or demonic forces. Spiritual suffering seems to be involved in the process of examining what is valued and how this informs life meaning, particularly when what is valued does not live up to one's expectations. This process may be reflected in and/or prompted by a combination of spiritual struggles.

Mako et al. (2006) applied the Pargament et al. (2005) framework in studying the experience of spiritual pain in patients with advanced-stage cancer. Each patient's description of spiritual pain was categorized based on being associated with interpersonal, intrapsychic (intrapersonal), and/or divine struggles. Forty-eight percent of patients identified with intrapsychic dimensions of spiritual pain. This domain included the widest range of emotions, including resignation and despair (40 percent), abandonment or isolation (20 percent), anxiety (10 percent), and regret (10 percent). Thirty-eight percent of patients described divine dimensions associated with spiritual pain. The emotions most associated with this domain were resignation and despair (32 percent), anxiety (28 percent), and isolation (8 percent). Thirteen percent of patients reported interpersonal dimensions of spiritual pain. This domain was characterized by feelings of isolation (71 percent) and regret (24 percent). The authors found a significant overlap between reports of spiritual pain and depression. Less than 30 percent of patients associated spiritual pain with physical symptoms such as generalized pain or ache in the heart. The presence and intensity of spiritual pain was consistent regardless of age, gender, religious affiliation, or level of religious involvement. However, Catholics were significantly less likely than individuals of other religious faiths to describe spiritual pain in terms of the divine and more likely to express their spiritual pain in terms of intrapsychic conflict. As in efforts used to measure physical pain, patients were asked to rate their intensity of spiritual pain on a scale from 0 to 11. Patient levels of spiritual pain ranged from 0.67 to 8.73, with an average score of 4.70.

It is hard to know exactly what this means, given that the experience of pain, including physical pain, is subjective (Draper, 2012). Nevertheless, however difficult it is to measure pain, evidence suggests that many patients have a unique experience of spiritual pain that has the potential to compromise biopsychosocial and spiritual functioning.

Potential Consequences

Given that there is some relationship between biopsychosocial and spiritual functioning, spiritual suffering can significantly reduce overall life quality (Balboni et al., 2007; Chochinov & Cann, 2005; Delgado-Guay et al., 2011; Edwards et al., 2010; Hebert, Zdaniuk, Schulz, & Scheier, 2009; Hills et al., 2005; HPNA, 2013; Mako et al., 2006; Pargament & Ano, 2006; Peteet & Balboni, 2013; Puchalski, 2008a, 2008c; Puchalski et al., 2006; Vallurupalli et al., 2011; Winkelman et al., 2011; Wynne, 2013; Yang et al., 2010). For example, spiritual suffering has been associated with poorer psychological adjustment and mental health (Balboni et al., 2007; Hebert et al., 2009; Pargament & Ano, 2006; Peteet & Balboni, 2013; Winkelman et al., 2011). Patients may refuse to accept having a terminal illness (Wynne, 2013; Yang et al., 2010). A lack of life meaning could provoke hopelessness, fear, powerlessness, and depression (Edwards et al., 2010; Hebert et al., 2009; Mako et al., 2006; Puchalski, 2008a; Yang et al., 2010). Social isolation can result in the absence of trusted others to share spiritual concerns and reduced involvement with family and community life (Edwards, et al., 2010; Langegard & Ahlberg, 2009; Murray et al., 2004; Pargament & Ano, 2006; Peteet & Balboni, 2013; Yang et al., 2010). Spiritual suffering can have negative implications for health, for example, it can entail an increased need for medical services and mortality risk (Chochinov & Cann, 2005; Edwards, et al., 2010; Hills et al., 2005; Mako et al., 2006; Pargament & Ano, 2006; Pargament et al., 2001; Puchalski, 2008c; Puchalski et al., 2006; Wynne, 2013), although research has been unable to consistently validate this relationship (Chochinov & Cann, 2005; Delgado-Guay et al., 2011; Mako et al., 2006; Pargament, Koenig, Tarakeshwar, & Hahn, 2001; Vallurupalli et al., 2011). Spiritual suffering can increase the risk that patients will engage in treatment noncompliance (Wynne, 2013). Therefore, spiritual suffering has the potential to affect one's entire being (HPNA, 2013). This reflects the importance of strategies that help patients prevent and/or reduce spiritual suffering as they cope with the dying process.

SPIRITUAL RESILIENCE

Although it may be difficult to identify spiritual suffering, hospice social workers should still be able to help patients mobilize resources for spiritual support. Mobilizing resources for spiritual support provides a proactive response to the dying process that may sustain and/or build spiritual resilience (Nakashima, 2007). Social work intervention may be necessary to help patients gain access to these spiritual resources. Part of this process is to draw from existing resources if not to discover new ones (Byock, 1996). As suggested in chapter 3, the approach will vary by patient relative to a patient's spiritual needs. Support may come from resources such as prayer, reading inspirational material, being with friends, listening to music, or seeking reconciliation. Researchers have found that reliance on such spiritual resources has the potential to help hospice patients enhance life quality (Ando et al., 2009; Brennan, 2013; Campbell & Ash, 2007; Johnson, 2011; Nakashima, 2007; Narayanasamy, 2007; Peteet & Balboni, 2013; Pevey, Jones, & Yarber, 2009; Sherburne, 2008; Smith et al., 2012; Tuck et al., 2012; Wynne, 2013). As seen in figure 4.1, Grant et al. (2004) suggested that the meeting of spiritual needs could prevent and/or reduce the potential for spiritual distress. Misunderstanding this potential relationship increases the risk for the utilization of health care interventions that fail to address underlying spiritual needs.

Grant et al. (2004) interviewed 20 patients (13 with advanced cancer and 7 with advanced nonmalignant illness) twice, 3 months apart in the last year of life. They asked the patients about their spiritual needs and the extent to which unmet spiritual needs impacted their overall well-being, including their need for resources for support. Spiritual needs were defined

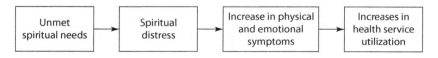

FIGURE 4.1   Possible effects of unmet spiritual needs.
Source: Grant et al. (2004).

as "the needs and expectations which humans have to find meaning, purpose and value in their life. Such needs can be specifically religious, but even people who have no religious faith or are not members of an organized religion have belief systems that give their lives meaning and purpose" (p. 372). Although two patients denied having spiritual needs, others expressed the need to search for meaning and identity, peace, and a guide into the unknown. Patients expressed a desire to search for meaning, particularly when they were diagnosed with terminal illness or when their symptoms incapacitated them. Patients said they felt useless and lacking in purpose as their roles within their families and larger life were displaced by illness. They wondered whether they were experiencing divine judgment or indifference. Patients indicated a desire for peace and, thus, freedom from the fear of death that seemed the most intense at night. Even though they said they knew doctors could provide medications to control physical symptoms, they wanted someone to help them face death. Their questions about the end of life became more specific when death seemed imminent. There were patients who were dismayed by how little support they received while in the process of dying in contrast to how much support they received when giving birth. Patients wanted a professional caregiver to help them understand what was happening to them. They wanted support, for example, through the provision of information and guidance.

Grant et al. (2004) also interviewed each patient's primary-care doctor to learn more. Based on these results, the authors determined that unmet spiritual needs could lead to spiritual distress. Spiritual distress was indicated by an increase in physical and emotional symptoms and more service utilization to cope (see figure 4.1). When service utilization failed to reduce spiritual distress, this led to continued suffering and more services that failed to address a patient's underlying spiritual needs. Although additional research is needed to test this model, hospice social workers can still be a proactive spiritual resource for patients. Terminal illness can challenge spiritual beliefs and practices and evoke intense emotions (Lukoff, n.d.; Puchalski, 2013; Thune-Boyle, Stygall, Keshtgar, & Newman, 2006). Grant et al. found that patients had the capacity to meet their own spiritual needs if given support:

> Some accepted the inevitability of death, and spoke of a universal allotted span of life. . . . Being able to talk about illness was important. . . . Many found meaning in family relationships. . . . Others adopted a resilient, almost

stoical approach. . . . Some found strength and hope in their beliefs and in the promise of a life after death, frequently interpreting their illness within their belief system. . . . Reading the Bible, meditating, attending religious services, or sitting in the garden brought comfort and reduced angst. Even some nonreligious patients found prayer therapeutic and some felt it lessened their physical pain.

(pp. 373–374)

Patients indicated that they coped best when they had the support of families and professionals. They talked about the desire to be treated as individuals, which helped them retain a sense of worth and meaning. Some even suggested a desire to engage in prayer with their professional caregivers, which inspired hope. Grant et al. (2004) said that "being treated as individuals who were important, rather than diseases, made the most difference to how people felt on a day-to-day basis" (p. 374). Social workers can be among those professionals who develop positive relationships with patients that reduce risk for spiritual suffering (Edwards et al., 2010). Therefore, having access to spiritual resources may reduce a patient's risk for spiritual suffering and increase life quality (Edwards, et al., 2010; Grant, et al., 2004; Hills et al., 2005; Lukoff, n.d.; Peteet, & Balboni, 2013).

Religious Coping

Negative religious coping, which would necessitate a referral to a spiritual caregiver, provides another example of how unmet spiritual needs can increase the risk for spiritual suffering. Thune-Boyle, Stygall, Keshtgar, and Newman (2006) conducted a systematic review of the literature on religious coping defined as "the use of cognitive and behavioural techniques, in the face of stressful life events, that arise out of one's religion or spirituality" (p. 152). It was difficult to draw firm conclusions, but the authors did report finding significant effects of self-defeating thoughts associated with negative religious coping (see box 4.1 for examples; Hebert et al., 2009). Some of the most notable work employed the RCOPE and Brief RCOPE measures developed by Pargament (2007) and associates (Pargament, Smith, Koenig, & Perez, 1998; Pargament, Feuille, & Burdzy, 2011). These measures are based on the theory that people use a combination of religious coping methods to deal with major life stressors. Methods of religious coping involved different thoughts, feelings, behaviors, and relationships. These methods were considered positive (adaptive) or negative (maladaptive) religious coping. Positive religious coping reflected a secure relationship with a supportive God, a sense of spiritual connection with others, and belief that life had meaning. Negative religious coping reflected a tenuous relationship with a punishing God, a threatening view of the world, and a struggle to find meaning.

Pargament, Smith, Koenig, and Perez (1998) tested the Brief RCOPE measure with three different populations, including 551 patients hospitalized due to a medical illness. They found that positive and negative religious coping methods were associated with different outcomes. People were more likely to rely on positive religious coping, which was linked to fewer symptoms of psychological distress and spiritual growth. Negative religious coping was associated with more symptoms of psychological distress and poorer quality of life. Negative religious coping was indicated by interpreting a stressful situation as God's punishment for sins, discontented relationships with congregational members or clergy relative to a stressful situation, questioning God's power to influence a stressful situation, interpreting a stressful situation as a demonic act, and a discontented relationship with God relative to a stressful situation (Pargament et al., 2011). The Brief RCOPE was further tested and reduced to seven items for each set of positive and negative religious coping methods as found in box 4.1. Although the authors did not test the Brief RCOPE on patients with terminal illness, subsequent studies have employed this measure and confirmed that negative religious coping is significantly related to lower life quality and life satisfaction (Balboni et al., 2007; Delgado-Guay et al., 2011; Hebert et al., 2009; Hills et al., 2005; Pargament, Koenig, Tarakeshwar, & Hahn, 2001; Vallurupalli et al., 2011).

Hebert, Zdaniuk, Schulz, and Scheier (2009) explored religious coping by surveying 189 women at stage I or II breast cancer and stage IV breast cancer at study entry and 8 to 12 months later. The authors explored relationships between positive and negative coping and depression, physical and psychological well-being, and life satisfaction. They measured religious coping by using four items from the RCOPE scale. The majority of women (76 percent) were likely to use at least a moderate amount of positive religious coping. A smaller proportion (15 percent) of patients reported using at least some negative religious coping. Negative religious coping, indicated

BOX 4.1   THE BRIEF RCOPE: POSITIVE AND NEGATIVE COPING
SUBSCALE ITEMS

Positive Religious Coping Subscale Items

1. Looked for a stronger connection with God
2. Sought God's love and care
3. Sought help from God in letting go of my anger
4. Tried to put my plans into action together with God
5. Tried to see how God might be trying to strengthen me in this situation
6. Asked forgiveness for my sins
7. Focused on religion to stop worrying about my problems

Negative Religious Coping Subscale Items

1. Wondered whether God had abandoned me
2. Felt punished by God for my lack of devotion
3. Wondered what I did for God to punish me
4. Questioned God's love for me
5. Wondered whether my church had abandoned me
6. Decided the devil made this happen
7. Questioned the power of God

Source: Pargament et al. (1998).

in some instances by expressing anger at God and wondering whether God had abandoned them, was significantly associated with the experience of depression, poor mental health, and less life satisfaction regardless of sociodemographics and other factors. These results were consistent with other studies that found negative religious coping was significantly related to psychological distress (Balboni et al., 2007; Pargament & Ano, 2006). Interestingly, this relationship did not vary based on cancer stage, so the relationships between negative religious coping and well-being factors were no different over time. That means a patient's coping style was constant regardless of change in health status or other factors. The one consolation, although not for some patients, was the low incidence of negative religious coping. This finding was supported by similar studies (Pargament et al., 1998, 2001; Ellison & Lee, 2010).

CONCLUSION

A terminal illness is the ultimate test of the human spirit (Pesut, 2008). Research shows that patients with terminal illness are at risk for spiritual suffering, although spiritual suffering may not be defined in the same way or experienced to the same degree (Byock, 1996; Chaturvedi, 2007; Exline et al., 2013; HPNA, 2013; Mako et al., 2006; Murray et al., 2004; Narayanasamy, 2007; Nixon & Narayanasamy, 2010; Peteet & Balboni, 2013; Puchalski, 2008a). Mako et al. (2006) found that 55 out of 57 patients interviewed with advanced-stage cancer experienced spiritual pain but described this experience in different ways. Spiritual suffering can have significant implications for overall life quality (Exline et al., 2013; HPNA, 2013; Mako et al., 2006; Murray et al., 2004; Nixon & Narayanasamy, 2010; Pargament & Ano, 2006; Peteet & Balboni, 2013; Puchalski, 2008a). Patients risk continued suffering due to fear, desire to protect others, or inability to describe the intangible aspects of their experience (Langegard & Ahlberg, 2009; Mako et al., 2006; Murray et al., 2004; Peteet & Balboni, 2013; Tan, Braunack-Mayer, & Beilby, 2005; Yang et al., 2010). Langegard and Ahlberg (2009) suggest these patients experience double suffering in the process. Alternatively, for some, spiritual suffering can lead to reliance on spiritual resources that enable relative comfort in the months, weeks, days, and hours before death (Byock, 1996; Narayanasamy, 2007; Pesut, 2008; Peteet & Balboni, 2013; Wynne, 2013).

Terminal illness interrupts normal life and affords the opportunity to embrace what is meaningful (Byock, 1996). The way a patient responds can transform the dying process into a spiritual process. Spiritual suffering may be one of the factors that moves patients to acknowledge losses as well as discover new meaning, redefine social roles and expectations, maintain self-esteem, and experience hope and inner peace (Narayanasamy, 2007; Nakashima, 2007; Puchalski, 2013; Thune-Boyle et al., 2006). For some, this experience entails reliance on spiritual resources to transcend spiritual suffering (Yang et al., 2010). As described by Cassell (1982):

Transcendence is probably the most powerful way in which one is restored to wholeness after an injury to personhood. When experienced, transcendence locates the person in a far larger landscape. The sufferer is not isolated by pain but is brought closer to a transpersonal source of meaning and to the human community that shares those meanings. Such an experience need not involve religion in any formal sense: however, in its transpersonal dimension, it is deeply spiritual.

(p. 644)

This is not to suggest that patient access to spiritual resources guarantees transcendence or that spiritual suffering can be avoided. Again, the experience of dying is as unique as each patient's experience of spirituality. Spirituality can be a significant resource or stressor depending on how each patient experiences the dying process. Hospice social workers can help patients draw from spiritual resources that validate personhood and proactively build and/or sustain spiritual resilience (Cassell, 1982). Chapter 5 addresses how hospice social workers can *be* one of those spiritual resources.

PART 2

Facilitating Quality Spiritual Care

5

Relational Spirituality

IT TAKES A SPECIAL PERSON to support another in the fullness of being human, particularly when being human includes feelings that are uncomfortable (Goldberg & Crespo, 2003). In the experience of hospice care, therapeutic relationships provide a formal way of connecting with a trained professional that can change one's life profoundly. Therapeutic relationships are not only necessary for a hospice social worker to ensure a patient's basic needs are met but also in providing other forms of care to support a patient's psychosocial and spiritual well-being. The gravity of facing a terminal illness places unique demands on the therapeutic relationship. Needs arise in patients, and perhaps in hospice social workers, that are unanticipated. Existential challenges associated with terminal illness can make an individual question his or her core beliefs and motivation to go on. Hence, within the context of hospice care, patients and social workers have the opportunity to experience a therapeutic relationship that can feel spiritual in nature. This chapter will explore how a therapeutic relationship may inform a hospice patient's experience of spirituality and ultimately serve as a spiritual resource.

DEFINING THERAPEUTIC RELATIONSHIPS

Central to the delivery of hospice social work are therapeutic relationships. Therapeutic relationships may last for a short time to months and years. They may involve telephone or face-to-face contact in a person's home, outpatient facility, or hospital unit (Priebe & McCabe, 2008). A therapeutic relationship may be defined as a relational process that involves thoughts, feelings, and behaviors at the core of an encounter (Saunders, 2001; Skovholt, 2005). This relational process provides the context for care. In the hospice environment, a therapeutic relationship is a partnership designed to promote optimum health (Canning et al., 2007). Although there is less research on the experience of hospice social workers, related research suggests that the therapeutic relationship is a critical component in the delivery of care, with significant implications for treatment outcomes (Canning et al., 2007; Feller & Cottone, 2003; Kim, Kim, & Boren, 2008; Priebe & McCabe, 2008; Skovholt, 2005). For example, in a study with 74 palliative-care nurses in Australia, Canning et al. (2007) found that clear professional boundaries reduced conflict, promoted patient empowerment, and improved treatment outcomes. Norcross (2012) reviewed a series of meta-analyses to investigate the association between the therapeutic (or therapy) relationship and treatment effectiveness. The author found "beneficial, medium-sized effects of several elements of the complex therapy relationship" (p. 2). These elements included therapeutic alliance, cohesion, empathy, goal consensus and collaboration, positive regard and affirmation, and congruence/genuineness. A therapeutic relationship may have an indirect effect on treatment effectiveness, for example, by encouraging treatment engagement and compliance, and a direct effect through the relational processes, which Priebe and McCabe (2008) said "may be seen as therapy in itself" (p. 521). A therapeutic relationship may likewise have significant implications for the effectiveness of hospice social work (Priebe & McCabe, 2008; Saunders, 2001).

CONDITIONS FOR A THERAPEUTIC RELATIONSHIP

Although there are many conditions associated with the provision of hospice care, the therapeutic relationship is one that can support treatment effectiveness. This requires hospice social workers to develop the qualities and skills necessary to cultivate a therapeutic style of engagement (Allamani, 2007; Chatters & Taylor, 2003; Feller & Cottone, 2003; Norcross, 2012; Priebe & McCabe, 2008; Saunders, 2001; Skovholt, 2005). Research across disciplines has consistently found that effective communication, positive emotional bond, agreement on treatment goals, and treatment collaboration help make a relationship therapeutic (Allamani, 2007; Canning et al.,

2007; Feller & Cottone, 2003; Horvath, Del Re, Flückiger, & Symonds, 2011; Norcross, 2012; Kim et al., 2008; Mok & Chiu, 2004). Palliative-care research further suggests that patients desire a therapeutic relationship that enables access to information, empowerment, shared goal setting and decision making, and respect for autonomy and diversity (Canning et al., 2007; Mok & Chiu, 2004). The therapeutic relationship has been particularly important to hospice- and palliative-care patients and their families (Canning et al., 2007).

In a qualitative study with 10 palliative-care nurses and their patients in China, Mok and Chiu (2004) found that patients were the most concerned about the quality of the therapeutic relationship. Patients sought therapeutic relationships that involved trust, security, and reciprocity. Similar qualities of empathy, positive regard, affirmation, and genuineness were identified as being significant in psychology research (Feller & Cottone, 2003; Norcross, 2012). Skovholt (2005) conducted a study of experienced psychotherapists and found that therapeutic qualities and skills fell under three domains: cognitive, emotional, and relational. The cognitive domain included flexibility to embrace ambiguity, understanding of the human condition, and appreciation of lifelong learning. The emotional domain included humility, self-awareness, and self-acceptance. The relational domain included keen interpersonal perception, capacity for intense engagement, and ability to express compassion. As described by Carl Rogers (2007), founder of the person-centered humanist approach, empathy is another essential quality that involves "feeling into" the experience of patients to sense their "private world as if it were your own, but without ever losing the 'as if' quality" (p. 243; Feller & Cottone, 2003).

Relational Depth

A therapeutic relationship provides an opportunity for patients to live in the world differently through experiences they have with hospice social workers (Berzoff, 2008). It is through "holistic listening" that hospice social workers allow themselves to deeply connect with their patients and discover the multifaceted aspects of their lives (Baker, 2005, p. 55; Knox, 2008). Likewise, as stated by Baker (2005), we are not only "in relationship with others, [but] we are also in relationship with the different aspects of ourselves" (p. 55). Hence, a therapeutic relationship can stimulate experiential learning and growth for patients *and* hospice social workers. Some degree of relational depth emerges relative to "the human need to be close, to be seen, to be known" (Baker, 2005, p. 55). As a result, the therapeutic relationship is a dynamic process of cocreation that informs the relational context of care (Baker, 2005; Knox, 2008). Although research on relational depth has focused on psychotherapeutic relationships, these findings may lend insight into therapeutic relationships developed through hospice social work.

Mearns (1997) introduced the concept of relational depth in counseling and psychotherapy research. Relational depth involves an enduring relationship with a high degree of empathy, congruence, and unconditional positive regard similar to the core conditions of growth involved in therapeutic presence (Baker, 2005; Knox, 2008; Knox, Murphy, Wiggins, & Cooper, 2013; Mearns, 2003; Mearns, Thorne, & McLeod, 2007; C. R. Rogers, 2007). As described by Cooper (2005), in relational depth the "inner spirit seems to reach out and touch the inner spirit of the other and she or he is closest to his or her 'inner, intuitive self,'" (p. 88). Mearns and Cooper (2005) further clarified by stating that relational depth is "a state of profound contact and engagement between two people, in which each person is fully real with the Other, and able to understand and value the Other's experiences at a high level" (p. xii). Relational depth is believed to influence treatment quality and outcomes, which may have implications for hospice social work (Baker, 2005; Cooper, 2005; Knox, 2008). How hospice social workers engage in care may likewise facilitate this experience of relational depth (Callahan, 2009b, 2012, 2013).

Based on Martin Buber's (1970) theory of dialogue, Callahan (2009b) suggested that an "I-Thou" and "I-It" style of communication are two different ways a hospice social worker might cultivate a therapeutic relationship. I-It communication is task oriented or instrumental in nature. It may be used to expedite care but is not described as an ideal mode of communication, for it risks objectifying a patient. I-Thou communication has the potential to validate the dignity and worth of a patient, congruent with social work professional ethics (NASW, 2008). Allamani (2007) described a similar style of engagement: "If the interaction is oriented more toward listening than just to find out solutions, disclosure about suffering may be allowed, and the persons may perceive that they are accepted as a whole, together with their disease. This lets an individual feel that that he/she is a human being and is part of a larger world: a positive cure is reached" (p. 234). Callahan (2009b, 2012, 2013) likewise described I-Thou communication as a mode of intervention that can be integrated throughout the provision of care (Canda & Furman, 1999, 2010). I-Thou communication entails qualities and skills that connote "spiritual sensitivity" (Callahan, 2009, p. 174). Although the application of I-Thou communication is largely generalist in nature, it can inform advanced generalist and clinical intervention relative to the expertise of the hospice social worker (Callahan, 2009, 2012, 2013). This process would likewise require professional boundaries to balance relational depth with detachment.

To further explore the emergence of relational depth, Cooper (2005) conducted a qualitative study with eight registered psychotherapists experienced in person-centered and existential practice. Cooper analyzed their responses, which where organized in three categories: self-experiences, perceptions of the client, and experiencing the relationship. Experiences of self during relational depth involved emotional states of intense empathy and deep acceptance of all aspects of the client. Therapists said they felt fully present, more authentic, and congruent with clients. There was an experience of an altered state of consciousness during which, for instance, they felt time had stopped. After the encounter, some therapists reported being energized or feeling lighter, while others felt drained. Unfortunately, the author did not explain why some therapists felt drained, but rather focused on the positive effects of relational depth. Therapists suggested a sense of rightness about the encounter that left them feeling optimistic for their clients. They believed that relational depth had led clients to new insights. Interestingly, one therapist said she realized such depth could only occur once she allowed herself to connect with her client and acknowledge that her client valued such a connection.

A follow-up qualitative study was conducted by Knox (2008) with 14 clients who had worked with person-centered psychotherapists. Clients were encouraged to discuss moments in which they did and did not experience relational depth with therapists. A couple of clients described moments of relational depth with supervisors. These accounts were also included in the study. Experiences of relational depth were described as having emerged through a deep connection with the self, therapist, and therapeutic relationship. Relational depth was also experienced as being fully present in the moment. There was a general consensus that the experience of relational depth was meaningful or powerful and had enduring effects. Clients reported feeling more energized, positive, confident, and at ease. Relational depth was said to have facilitated healing within and had a positive effect on the therapeutic relationship. The experience of relational depth also facilitated an enduring feeling of validation. Some were better able to respond to later challenges and improve other relationships.

Professional Boundaries

In cultivating a therapeutic relationship, hospice social workers must negotiate the paradox of being "emotionally involved yet emotionally distant, united but separate," for they are at risk for "caring too much" in encountering another's pain (Skovholt, 2005, p. 88). According to Skovholt, this may require "boundaried generosity" to regulate deep engagement with patients (p. 88). Professional boundaries help hospice social workers remain in touch with professional roles and responsibilities. It is this ability to negotiate professional boundaries that helps hospice social workers sustain the capacity to care over and over again (Faver, 2004). Hospice social workers may employ Buber's (1970) I-Thou style of engagement and/or create the conditions for relational depth in effort to cultivate a therapeutic relationship, but they must balance connection with detachment for healthy relationship maintenance. For example, hospice social workers need to understand the extent to which patients are comfortable with the experience of relational depth. There may be other ways of cultivating a therapeutic relationship that are less intense and more spiritually sensitive, congruent with a patent's comfort level. Therefore, in the process of cultivating a therapeutic relationship, hospice social workers must continuously assess patient needs and their response to care to ensure that the therapeutic relationship ultimately serves as a vehicle for spiritually sensitive hospice social work.

WHEN RELATIONSHIPS INFORM SPIRITUALITY

The experience of relating that enhances life meaning is one of the many ways to define spirituality, as introduced in chapter 2 (MacConville, 2006; Weatherby, 2002). According to Heyse-Moore (1996), "we exist to relate to each other and if we do not our spirit dries up within us like a desert" (p. 307). Relationships can inform life meaning, which includes the need to build and/or sustain spiritual resilience. Eisenhandler (2005) interviewed 46 older adults and found that they described spirituality as being shaped by relationships both past and present. For respondents who lived in long-term care facilities, this involved relationships with professionals called "faithreps" (p. 85). Faithreps were said to have facilitated opportunities for faith expression that, for instance, involved talking about daily life and life's meaning. Eisenhandler concluded that spiritual awareness was a powerful force that helped these older adults find new ways of experiencing life as it unfolded, but it required one to move to an enlarged sense of self, sense of others, and sense of life as a whole. This included a desire to engage in relationships made possible through one's environment. The process of engaging in relationships informed a spirituality that was dynamic in nature as it evolved over time. Hence, connectedness gave these older adults a sense of life meaning that was experienced as spirituality (Edser & May, 2007).

Other authors have described spirituality as an "innate human yearning for meaning through intra-, inter-, and transpersonal connectedness" (Belcher and Griffiths, 2005, p. 272; Bullis, 1996; Canda, 1999; Hermann, 2001; Sandage & Shults, 2007; Staude, 2005; Wright, 2002). Western and Eastern religions emphasize practices that involve cultivating spiritual relationships within the self and/or with something outside the self, such as other people, the environment, or a divine higher power (Larimore, Parker, & Crowther, 2002). For example, a central focus in Christianity is to cultivate an intimate relationship with God that magnifies love for self and others and inspires actions that preserve God's creation. It is this pattern of relationships that "give[s] meaning and coherence to the way individuals understand the unfolding of their lives" (Stephenson, Draucker, & Martsolf, 2003, p. 51). From this perspective, "all spirituality can be viewed as relational" (Sandage & Shults, 2007, p. 263), since people are "beings-in relationship" (Sulmasy, 2002, p. 24). If spirituality is informed by meaning that unfolds through relationships, then relationships must be entered for spirituality to be understood, even if only partially (Stanworth, 2006). Therefore, it helps to explore how hospice patients may experience spirituality through connecting within, with others, and with the environment.

Connecting Within

Spirituality has been described as an interior process that involves conscious awareness and integration of observations (Egan et al., 2011; Hay, 2000; Sandage & Shults, 2007; Schneiders, 2003). This experience of spirituality may occur in response to how people understand their place within the larger world, which suggests a basic spiritual need for relationships that inform life meaning and purpose. Hay (2000) describes the awareness of this spiritual need for meaningful relationships as "relational consciousness." Considering hospice patients are likely to have different levels of spiritual self-awareness, it is reasonable to assume that relational consciousness would also lie on a continuum. Some hospice patients might be more consciously aware of the spiritual need for meaningful relationships. They may also have different levels of need for meaningful relationships and different concepts of what defines a meaningful relationship. Nevertheless, Hay suggests that a degree of relational consciousness is required to motivate efforts to cultivate and maintain relationships that build community, including a spiritual community. Thwarting relational consciousness can ultimately damage community connectedness. Only the individual can recognize the degree to which relationships are necessary to inform life meaning and thus realize the potential to experience relational spirituality. This insight requires a level of relational consciousness, which necessitates a connection with the self for spiritual self-awareness.

A study by Egan et al. (2011) further reflects how a connection with the self can define the experience of define spirituality. The study included 52 semistructured interviews and a survey of 642 hospice patients, family members, and staff in New Zealand. The authors collected a variety of responses that were organized into three categories: religious, existential/humanist, and summative. Specific to patients and family members, the majority of their responses fell under the existential/humanistic category. Relational/integration/wholeness was a related subcategory. Integration was described in relational terms that suggested being connected to a sense of self, feeling a part of things outside the self, and/or identifying with a place of origin allowed for spiritual wholeness. There were other subcategories that reflected the spiritual importance of cultivating a relationship with the self. For example, as part of the subcategory of core/essence/identity/well-being, some respondents said spirituality was defined by one's core self, known only to the person. This was likely to be illuminated through mindfulness, which was identified as a separate subcategory. Therefore, it seemed a relationship with the self was necessary to seek interior alignment with some perceived reality. This allowed for a sense of wholeness that motivated positive engagement in the world and spiritual resilience to create new meaning in the face of life challenges.

One of the most direct examples of how spirituality can emerge in the process of connecting with the self can be observed through spiritual and/or religious expression. In the previously mentioned study by Egan et al. (2011), respondents also identified internal states such as mindfulness in defining spirituality. This implied that a particular internal state might also serve as a way to experience spirituality. Perhaps mindfulness was used to heighten one's spiritual awareness for spiritual growth and/or for coping with terminal illness. Although the relationship is complex, there are many studies on health and mental health care that support the therapeutic effects of spiritual and/or religious coping (Van Hook & Rivera, 2004). For example, Goldstein (2007) conducted a study on individuals who were randomly assigned to a 3-week treatment group instructed on how to cultivate sacred moments or a control group instructed on how to write therapeutically about daily activities. The treatment was considered equally effective as the control based on improvements in spiritual well-being, psychological well-being, stress level, and daily spiritual experiences. The author found that these improvements were sustained over time when measured at 3 weeks and again at 6 weeks. Although this particular study does not focus on patients with terminal illness, it does reflect how a meaningful connection with the self provides a way to experience spirituality. What is not clear is the extent to which this experience of spirituality is bound by the limits of one's capacity for self-awareness.

Connecting with Others

The experience of connecting with others may also facilitate the experience of spirituality for hospice patients. Again, as social beings, it is through relationships with other human beings that people are able to populate the world. People serve as companions, protectors, and mentors, starting with one's primary caregiver. It is in relation to one's primary caregiver that ideas about the world originate that can last a lifetime. From a psychological standpoint, the self-in-relation theory involves seeing one's self in relation to people with whom one engages. Relationships can help inform one's sense of identity and build self-confidence and self-worth. The process of relating also provides the opportunity to experience mutual empathy, intimacy, and conflict resolution (Warwick, 2001). Such relationships and the quality of the relational experience can be what informs life meaning and, thus, a spiritual experience through connections with others. Spiritual or religious leaders may be among those with whom patients relate. They can provide inspiration for hospice patients when hope dims, and clarify ways to seek transcendence. They too may serve as proxies for the divine when patients need spiritual healing (Warwick, 2001). Object relations theory would suggest that all relationships involve transference and so provide a means of addressing internalized conflicts. Seeing how patients project (or express) their feelings about a higher power in relationships may lend powerful insight into a patient's experience of spirituality and potential for growth (Hall, 2004; S.A. Rogers, 2007).

Tan et al. (2005) conducted a qualitative study with 12 hospice patients receiving inpatient care to learn more about how they expressed spirituality and the impact of the hospice environment. Patients reported a reliance on uplifting things (i.e., music, nature, humor), spiritual practices (i.e., prayer, meditation, forgiveness), and having hope (i.e., from spiritual beliefs, of finding meaning). Some of these forms of spiritual expression could be accomplished independently. However, respondents also stressed the importance of relationships as an outlet for spiritual expression. Relationships with others allowed patients to retain a sense of life meaning. They said family and friends kept them from feeling abandoned. They gained support that facilitated a sense of normalcy as they talked about daily life and mutual interests. Patients also reported that care providers helped create a hospice environment that supported spiritual expression. Conversely, not every encounter was described as being positive. One respondent described working with a care provider who seemed to be having problems at home. Clearly both positive and negative qualities of relationships can have implications for a patient's experience of spirituality.

Another way a relationship with others can shape a patient's experience of spirituality is through group work. It is in this context that hospice patients may gain valuable support from those who can identify with having a terminal illness. Group work may not be appropriate for all hospice patients, given medical complications and late hospice referral, but it can be used therapeutically to help patients experience spirituality. Miller et al. (2005) tested a 12-month intervention that provided participants the opportunity to learn about the psychosocial and spiritual aspects of living well while dying. Study participants were randomly assigned to a treatment group or a control group. The control group consisted of quarterly mailings about self-help resources and a phone call from the program coordinator to verify receipt. The treatment group met monthly and focused on information sharing to help reduce spiritual, psychological, and death-related distress. Control and treatment group baseline and posttest scores from a number of standardized measures were compared. There was evidence that the treatment group reduced depressive symptoms, reduced death-related feelings of meaningless, and increased spiritual well-being. The authors further suggested that the amount of exposure to the intervention ("dose" effect) seemed to improve outcomes, particularly for spiritual well-being. Significant outcomes could be explained by clinical intervention, as the group was educational in nature, led by a nonlicensed therapist, and relied on group members for peer support. It therefore seems that relationships with others can support hospice patients psychosocially and spiritually.

Connecting with the Environment

Zapf (2008) noted that social work researchers often describe spirituality as a characteristic of a person, such as whether a person is religious or spiritual or has a religious affiliation. Social work interventions are expected to be sensitive to a patient's spiritual and/or religious worldview, but Zapf contends that spirituality is more than that. Likewise, within the context of this book, spirituality is not considered a static quality but rather a dynamic process that is experiential in nature. It is through the experience of meaningful relationships that relational spirituality becomes a partial product of operating within the world. This experience includes connecting with the nonhuman world and the physical environment. So, to understand how hospice patients experience relational spirituality *in* the environment, hospice social workers must consider how patients experience spirituality *with* the environment (Zapf, 2008). Patients may not want to connect with the nonhuman world and the physical environment, but do want to connect with their treatment environment. For example, hospice care within a patient's home is likely to help that patient gain comfort through the familiar in a way that being in a sterile hospital room cannot.

Although more research is needed to validate the importance of a spiritually supportive environment, one account by Gregory and Gregory (2004) describes how one patient's ability to connect with something from nature helped facilitate the dying process. A patient's family member used a feather to empower the patient to mark her journey:

> The younger sister then, with pain in her heart and a lump in her throat, spoke: "Older sister, one of my friends knew I was coming to see you for," and here she whispered, "for the last time. This special friend gave me a gift to share with you. This gift, a feather, is to provide a safe journey to the spirit world." She embraced her older sister's hands with her own and gently placed the feather into her sister's hand, so she could feel and hold it. The younger sister added, "I give you this feather now, so when the time comes, you will be able to fly to the beyond, to where your spirit seeks to go. . . ." Family members gathered by the bedside and she looked for the last time at her younger sister and whispered, "Thank you for my feather, I am ready to fly now." While holding the feather tightly, she managed one last smile. That smile again filled the younger sister with hope and the knowledge that her older sister had been and would always be a part of who she was. At the burial, the woman's hands still embraced the feather. That evening, a feather-like shooting star streaked across the night sky, and the younger sister smiled.
>
> (p. 298)

This feather provided a natural bridge for this patient to move from the physical world to a spiritual world. Hence, by holding a feather, this patient was able to symbolize that accepting life meant accepting death. The patient, family, staff, and volunteers all worked together to make this possible. This also allowed the patient's loved ones time to prepare, experience, and grieve.

Hospice social workers can work to ensure hospice care is delivered in a spiritually supportive environment (Canda & Furman, 1999, 2010). As indicated in the previous study by Tan et al. (2005), hospice patients relied on relationships and held onto what was considered uplifting, engaged in spiritual practices, and maintained hope to express themselves spiritually. Hospice policies, staffing, programming, atmosphere, and physical environment were referenced as having some influence over patients' spiritual expression. Examples of spiritually supportive policies allowed for flexible visiting hours or no visitation if desired by the patient. Patients also noted the importance of having the option of a single room. They considered hospice providers who communicated care and compassion, humor and hope, and desire to listen and empower as being supportive of spiritual expression. Patients expressed the importance of worshipping as they pleased without fear of evangelization but also appreciated opportunities for interdenominational worship. There was a desire for an atmosphere of peace and quiet. The physical environment that was said to be spiritually supportive included having access to a variety of music, gardens, and pets to visit. Respondents also noted the importance of having access to adequate space to entertain larger groups. What is spiritually supportive is relative to each patient, but there are many ways hospice social workers can help.

As noted by Hall (2004), "People are fundamentally motivated by, and develop in the context of emotionally significant relationships" (p. 68). Relationships can have spiritual dimensions that are often not named (McGrath & Newell, 2004). The spiritual importance of relationships may be especially true for hospice patients. Terminal illness, like other life passages, provides an opportunity for new relational experiences that facilitate spiritual growth. Rather than relying on words, spirituality may be best understood through experience. For hospice patients, relationships provide a way to respond to "the human need to transcend, to go beyond the suffering and to find meaning in that experience" (Kellehear, 2000, p. 153). Relationships with self and others may inform one's spiritual identity and promote shared healing through group work. Cultivating an awareness of one's connection with the environment may be just as important. There is still much to learn about how relationships inform spirituality. The implications of such may likewise vary based on, for example, the degree of a patient's relational consciousness. However, the spiritual importance of relationships may not be a value that is recognized by all (Pesut, 2003). This suggests a need for a social work intervention model that explains how the therapeutic relationship may factor into the provision of spiritually sensitive hospice social work (Callahan, 2009, 2012, 2013; Sandage & Shults, 2007).

THE SPIRITUAL IMPORTANCE OF THERAPEUTIC
RELATIONSHIPS

Human beings operate through relationships that involve the experience of connection within, with others, and with the environment. Some of these relationships take on spiritual significance, as they inform the experience of life meaning and purpose. According to Davis, Hook, and Worthington (2008), "A relational definition of spirituality emphasizes that spirituality is contextualized within the fabric of a person's relationships" (p. 294). The types of relationships a person values reveals what is considered sacred and how one experiences the sacred. Sacred relationships may or may not include a formal religious affiliation, as the nature of relationships and their importance are relative to each person. However, some relationships may become sacred when faced with terminal illness. There are old and new relationships that may emerge as central to the experience of life meaning. One of these relationships might be the therapeutic relationship. Given the centrality of therapeutic relationships in hospice social work, the concept of relational spirituality can be used to inform the provision of care (Callahan, 2013, 2015; Faver, 2004; Krieglstein, 2006; Seyfried, 2007). Faver (2004) first described the concept of relational spirituality in a qualitative study of 50 service providers and advocates. This concept was later extended by Callahan (2012b, 2015) to apply to hospice social workers.

Based on the work of feminist philosopher Carol Ochs (1986, 1997), Faver (2004) said relationships are an opportunity to "complement, challenge, and expand" one's own perspective but requires a willingness to grow (p. 242; Krieglstein, 2006; Seyfried, 2007). The process of providing social work was believed to allow for interdependence to occur between a care provider and care receiver. It was this type of relationship that was said to reflect a more inclusive, loving reality that involved fully appreciating the reality of the other. This type of relationship also required receptivity to being open and authentic, similar to Buber's (1970) I-Thou communication, rather than a false projection of the self, more congruent with I-It communication. As further described by Faver (2004), "This connection is a spiritual dimension of helping" (p. 248). It is this connection that enlarged a caregiver's capacity to care so much so that the process of caregiving magnified the joy of the caregiver. Faver found

that this type of care facilitated a "joy and vitality" that went beyond satisfaction with outcomes (p. 243). It was suggested that the joy of relating not only sustained the caregiving relationship but also enhanced the
spiritual capacity to sustain care, as it provided renewal for the caregiver.
Otis-Green (2006) seemed to reflect this experience:

> Soul work invites introspection. I often say that a diagnosis of cancer is an
> invitation to consider the possibility of one's own mortality. Now I recog-
> nize that to work with those with a life-threatening illness also invites the
> attentive caregiver to consider the same. In this role, we have the privilege
> to see dying done by experts, and to benefit from this vicarious learning
> opportunity. What I have learned is that regrets increase our suffering, and
> that dying comes packaged with enough suffering without adding any more.
> I have tried to use that knowledge in guiding my decision making ever since.
> I have discovered that despite the challenges inherent in identifying oneself
> as a "change-agent," the rewards are greater still. I sleep better at night know-
> ing that I have tried to take a stand and make a difference. Sitting at the
> bedside of a dying person reminds me that our work matters.
>
>   (pp. 1477–1478)

Callahan (2015) described this spirituality of relatedness "as the experience of enhanced life meaning through a morally fulfilling relationship with the self, someone/something else, or higher power" (p. 49).
Callahan (2013, 2015) suggested that hospice social workers could cultivate
the experience of relational spirituality through a spiritually sensitive style
of caregiving. This style of caregiving has the potential to validate a patient's
inherent dignity and worth and enhance a patient's experience of life meaning. A patient's perception of enhanced life meaning through the therapeutic relationship was described as the experience of relational spirituality,
which was said to confirm a therapeutic relationship as being spiritually
sensitive. In a qualitative study on hospice-care providers, Callahan (2013)
found that the communication of spiritual sensitivity included particular
qualities and skills, such as recognizing personhood, therapeutic touch,
being present, listening, singing, reframing, affirming, self-disclosure,
normalization, and advocacy. It was suggested that a spiritually sensitive
style of engagement could be a form of spiritual care insofar that it facilitated the experience of relational spirituality, thus making the therapeutic

relationship *itself* a therapeutic intervention. Therefore, combining this with previous research, relational spirituality can be defined by relationships that are growth producing in that they inform life meaning, which strengthens one's capacity to care.

Psychological Process Models

Other scholars in nursing and psychology have described relational spirituality based on psychological processes (Davis, Worthington, Hook, & Tongeren, 2009; S.A. Rogers, 2007; Sandage & Williamson, 2010; Simpson, Newman, & Fuqua, 2008; Stern & James, 2006). Relational spirituality is considered the product of internalized relational schemas. These relational schemas are believed to inform how to reconcile developmental and existential challenges and thus stimulate psychological growth and sense of life meaning. Simpson, Newman, and Fuqua (2008) conducted a study on Christians and found internalized relational models appeared to shape expectations and behaviors in a variety of relationships. They suggested this internalized schema influenced relationships on both the horizontal (with others) and vertical (with the divine) levels. The authors likewise found that measures of vertical relational dimensions accounted for 35 percent of the variance in measures of horizontal relational dimensions. They suggested that, for example, how one related to the divine correlated with how one related to others and vice versa. This type of relationship was also found in research on forgiveness conducted by Davis et al. (2009). Simpson et al. (2008) conjectured that it was through these internalized relational schemas that religious practices could improve emotional health.

Hall (2004) developed a model of implicit relational representations to explain how relational spirituality might operate on the psychological level. This model is based on neuroscience and psychological theories such as multiple code theory, attachment theory, and object relations theory. Hall described five central principles associated with the implicit relational representations model as follows:

> *Central Organizing Principle #1.* People are fundamentally motivated by, and develop in the context of emotionally significant relationships. . . . Relationships provide the context of being for humans, or stated differently, the context for being human.

Central Organizing Principle #2. There are multiple codes of emotional information processing which provide a theoretical framework for understanding the way in which close relationships are processed and internalized, thereby shaping the patterns of our relationships with God, self and others.

Central Organizing Principle #3. Implicit relational representations are repetitions of relational experiences, sharing a common affective core, that are conceptually encoded in the mind as non-propositional meaning structures. They are the memory basis for implicit relational knowledge; that is, our "gut-level" sense of how significant relationships work.

Central Organizing Principle #4. Implicit relational representations, formed particularly from experiences in early relationships with caregivers, shape the emotional appraisal of meaning and subsequent patterns of relationship.

Central Organizing Principle #5. Implicit relational representations and knowledge form the foundation of our knowledge of self and others because they are processed automatically, and are not under the direct control of knowledge in the form of words that is processed in a linear manner.

(pp. 68–73)

In short, these principles suggest that relationships are necessary for survival. Patterns of relating within the self and/or with something outside of the self, such as other people, the environment, or a divine higher power are based on early relationships, starting with one's primary caregiver. These patterns are neurologically processed and become internalized, such that means of future relational patterns are implicitly understood and reactions are automatic.

Implications for Practice

The ways in which relationships inform spirituality are not clear-cut given the potential for spiritual diversity, but it does seem that relationships can inform spirituality and spirituality can inform relationships. Since relationships are central to hospice social work and have the potential to inform life meaning for patients, it is important to examine how the therapeutic relationship may be a spiritual resource in the context of hospice care. A hospice social worker can cultivate a spiritually sensitive relationship that supports patients' spiritual expression and enables them to meet their spiritual needs that build and/or sustain spiritual resilience (Gregory & Gregory, 2004; Mount, Boston, & Cohen, 2007; Olthuis, 1994). This would lead to the experience of enhanced life meaning, and thus relational spirituality. But before going on to further application, it is best to begin with examples of what relational spirituality might look like in practice.

Nursing research has contributed significantly in clarifying what it means to care spiritually. Penman et al. (2013) conducted in-depth interviews to explore what spiritual engagement meant from the perspective of four Australian palliative-care patients and 10 caregivers. Although this study did not include staff, the quality of spiritual engagement seemed to be supportive of relational spirituality. Spiritual engagement involved recognizing a patient's need to find life meaning while coping with a terminal illness. The key was caring for and being cared for by another. Everyday interactions were said to be supportive, as described here:

> Spiritual engagement pertains to intimate interactions where the client and caregiver not only revealed their spirituality to each other, but in a conversational context sought opportunities to share their innermost thoughts, beliefs, fears and vulnerabilities. The personal sharing of spiritual conversations usually took place when the relationship was deep, trusting and loving. When clients and caregivers shared their spirituality, they typically did so by sharing some account of what it meant for them, how they felt about it and why they engaged in spirituality.
>
> (p. 44)

Patients and caregivers both considered spiritual engagement a valuable resource and discussed similar qualities when describing the meaning of spiritual engagement. Spiritual engagement was said to involve maintaining relationships; participating in religious practice; human values of love, compassion, and altruism; personal transformation; and culture. Examples of distinct actions associated with spiritual engagement were showing and receiving love, praying, and participating in other religious practices. The authors suggested that such relationships should be cultivated in effort to support good spiritual care. Penman et al. concluded that:

> Terminal illness often creates suffering which precipitates spirituality for some individuals. Spirituality becomes real and important because it

empowers them to cope with their illness. The meaningfulness of suffering, impending death and heightened spirituality brings about personal transformation . . . [that] alters perceptions about self and others, and behaviour. The transforming experience affects sense of self and challenges the participants' thinking processes. . . . The change in character and action enabled clients and caregivers to be more loving and caring, patient and sacrificing for the "other."

(p. 44)

This experience was further described as "compassionate love" (p. 45). This type of love focuses on supporting what is good for another and, in doing so, helping that person feel understood. There was an emphasis on spiritual engagement in all types of relationships. Religion and culture were also identified as factors that shaped one's understanding of illness and provided an outlet for spiritual expression. It was expected that these relational spheres would interact and have different dynamics. Hence, this model seems to suggest that the experience of relational spirituality would be relative to the type and quality of relationships.

The previously mentioned qualitative study by Mok and Chiu (2004) with 10 palliative-care nurses and their patients in China lends more insight into what appears to be the experience of relational spirituality. The authors said that efforts to make the dying process meaningful were an integral part of the healing process, as patients often felt fearful, helpless, and lonely. Nurses communicated care through attitude and action. Being understanding and responsive helped cultivate a trusting relationship with patients. Understanding patient needs enabled nurses to advocate for their patients. This led patients to consider nurses as extended family members who were genuinely interested in them. The therapeutic relationship served as a means of enhancing inner strength for both patients and nurses. Patients drew from nurses as an outlet for expressing pain, a resource to finding peace, and incentive for going on. Even though these relationships focused on patient needs, nurses found their lives were enriched as well. Nurses were inspired by the way patients transcended their suffering. The therapeutic relationship ultimately evolved into one that facilitated mutual feelings of affection, trust, and connectedness. This positive relationship was central to achieving mutually agreed upon treatment goals. Hospice social workers have the potential to do the same.

The last example is a case study by McGrath and Newell (2004) that explores the spiritual life of one Australian woman in the last stages of Friedreich's ataxia. This disease had left her with minimal verbal skills, but the interview captured a rich relationship between her and her caregiver days before she passed away. It was the strong bonds of social support that seemed to inform her experience of spirituality. Throughout the progression of the disease, meaning making was centered on maintaining autonomy and living life with the help of others. The patient's connection with her caregiver was said to be on a deep, intuitive level. The caregiver offered physical support during the interview that conveyed a sense of comfort despite what the author described as "frightening symptoms [of the patient] . . . such as continually needing to gasp for breath" (p. 92). The caregiver communicated for the patient and validated her accuracy through nonverbal communication with the patient. For the caregiver, the process of providing patient care gave her inner satisfaction, although having limited access to supportive services made the process more burdensome. Nevertheless, this relationship provided a meaningful way to engage in and sustain the fullness of life, much like the experience of relational spirituality.

CONCLUSION

The purpose of hospice care is to reduce patient suffering and maximize comfort. Hospice social workers are available to help patients process the gravity of their condition. Complex emotions, thoughts, and behaviors left unaddressed can lead to suffering that includes spiritual suffering. The therapeutic relationship is an essential resource in delivering hospice social work and may also serve as a spiritual resource. Life quality necessitates relationships that are meaningful. This helps patients build and/or sustain spiritual resilience. The experience of life meaning gained through relationships suggests spiritual resilience is possible through relational spirituality. This allows for the therapeutic relationship to be a spiritual resource relative to the context of care. As observed by Mok and Chiu (2004), therapeutic engagement involves a series of negotiations that require caregiver commitment and patient trust for a mutually satisfactory relationship. The manner in which this process unfolds is relative to many factors, such as a patient's medical condition, feelings of vulnerability, and access to support, some of which cannot be controlled. However, a hospice social worker *can* employ therapeutic qualities and skills and exercise professional boundaries in effort to cultivate a spiritually sensitive relationship. This process involves a style of communication that allows for relational depth to emerge moderated by professional boundaries and patient comfort with the engagement. Hospice social workers must be spiritually sensitive to create a therapeutic space for this process to unfold. In the process, this increases the potential for hospice social workers and their patients to experience a meaningful relationship, and, thus, relational spirituality. The next chapter will examine how spiritually sensitive hospice social workers may facilitate the delivery of spiritual care.

6

Spiritual Care

SPIRITUAL CARE HAS BEEN AN essential part of end-of-life care since the founding of the hospice movement. National and international regulatory bodies require a spiritual assessment, but Medicare stipulations have not required hospice organizations to employ board-certified chaplains (BCCs) (Condition of Participation, 2010; Egan et al., 2011). This means other spiritual caregivers and interdisciplinary team members have shared in this work, leading to some debate over what denotes spiritual care, which hospice providers are qualified to provide spiritual care, and whether spiritual care should be eligible for insurance reimbursement (Glasper, 2011; Wright, 2002). Attempts have been made in research across disciplines to define spiritual care, but this process has been difficult (Daaleman et al., 2008). Perhaps this has been due, in part, to the many experiences of spirituality and different theoretical approaches used to inform how best to address spiritual needs. This chapter will define spiritual care by exploring the purpose of spiritual care, models for spiritual-care delivery, and patient reactions to receiving spiritual care. The chapter concludes with a relational model that demonstrates how spiritually sensitive hospice social work may serve as a form of spiritual care.

DEFINING SPIRITUAL CARE

Researchers across disciplines have asked what spiritual care means to hospice providers and patients (Egan et al., 2011). Nursing researchers have found that spiritual care has been considered a natural extension of biopsychosocial care (Carroll, 2001; Pesut, 2008b; Pike, 2011; Walter, 2002). This may allow for seamless integration of spiritual care into the delivery of hospice care but can be problematic when it is provided without being recognized as such (Pesut, 2008a, 2008c). As described by Touhy, Brown, and Smith (2005), the inability to distinguish spiritual care from other aspects of hospice care make it difficult to evaluate. Pesut (2008a) further suggested that being more intentional about delivering spiritual care as a distinct aspect of hospice care ensures spiritual care is based on assessment and outcomes associated with spiritual care delivery are evaluated. Training is needed to ensure spiritual care is provided relative to one's level of expertise and/or appropriate referrals are made to support the provision of spiritual care patients prefer. For hospice social workers, this process begins with clarifying the definition of spiritual care. Pesut (2008a) defined spiritual care relative to monism, theism, and humanism. One or more of these perspectives may be congruent with a patient's worldview. Hospice social workers can use this information to inform the purpose of spiritual care and associated activities.

Building on Pesut's work, a *monistic* perspective suggests that spiritual care is based on the assumption that all things and people are spiritually connected. Awareness of this universal connection may involve the dissolution of perceptual boundaries, so a patient feels a part of something larger than the self. This may be indicated by a suspension of space and time. Spiritual care focuses on enhancing a patient's awareness of spiritual transcendence over the limits of terminal illness through spiritual activities such as meditation or being outdoors. A *theistic* perspective suggests spiritual care is intended to help patients not only experience a universal connection but gain opportunities to seek a transcendent connection with a divine higher power. Spiritual care must respect a patient's religious beliefs and may involve spiritual activities such as engaging in religious rites or worship. This form of spiritual care may be more congruent with religious care, and a referral to a formal spiritual-care provider would be required. A *humanistic* perspective suggests spiritual care involves creating the conditions for patients to experience an awareness of life meaning and purpose. Spiritual care involves spiritual activities that support the subjective process of integrating new meaning, which may extend to the desire to engage in practices that facilitate transcendence or a religious experience. This may also include a therapeutic relationship that helps patients create (or perhaps cocreate) life meaning as a form of spiritual care.

Spiritual care has traditionally fallen under the auspices of formal spiritual-care providers such as hospice chaplains. As described in chapter 1, BCCs have the training to draw from a variety of spiritual-care perspectives based on the spiritual needs of patients (APC, 2004a, 2015a, 2015b). Chaplains can facilitate or ensure patient access to religious rites such as the administration of religious sacraments and prayer that is congruent with a theistic perspective and can employ supportive counseling skills such as active listening to help patients search for life meaning congruent with a humanistic perspective (Garces-Foley, 2006 Wright, 2002). Garces-Foley (2006) expressed concern that spiritual care has become less theistic and more humanistic over time as spiritual caregivers have changed. For example, when Medicare guidelines were established in 1982, hospices were required to address spiritual needs and document spiritual care but funds were not allocated. The Joint Commission further required spiritual care by a qualified professional but did not require this professional to be a BCC. Along with broader social trends, this has led to a more humanistic understanding of spirituality and a "psychologizing" of spiritual care (Garces-Foley, 2006, p. 125). For example, nursing-care plans are designed to address spiritual distress and cultivate spiritual well-being with the application of spiritual practices for spiritual coping (Ackley, Ladwig, & Makic, 2017). Spiritually integrated psychotherapy (Pargament, 2007) and spiritually sensitive hospice social work (Callahan, 2013) present alternative ways to provide spiritual care. Therefore, as spiritual-care providers have changed, so has the nature of spiritual care. Hospice social workers are among those who can facilitate the delivery of quality spiritual care if not directly by referral. In particular, a referral is necessary for the delivery of religious care because this is beyond the scope of hospice social work.

According to Gordon and Mitchell (2004), religious care is defined as care "given in the context of the shared religious beliefs, values, liturgies and lifestyle of a faith community" (p. 646). Spiritual care is defined as care "given in a one-to-one relationship, is completely person centred and makes no assumptions about personal conviction or life orientation" (p. 646). Religious care and spiritual care may overlap depending on patient needs and professional expertise of the spiritual-care provider (Driscoll, 2001; Glasper, 2011; Gordon & Mitchell, 2004; MacConville, 2006). As observed by Wright (2002), for some patients: "Spiritual care is a response to the requirements of faith. Consequently, it needs to be sensitive to the impact of those requirements upon daily life, and sympathetic to both religious and cultural traditions. This is particularly true where patients are separated from their faith community and dislocated from their normal pattern of daily life" (p. 130). Although spiritual care may focus on addressing existential issues associated with the dying process, spiritual-care providers must consider the potential for underlying religious issues and ensure religious care is provided by referral. Narrow adherence to any one perspective or approach can lead to neglect of patient needs and pressure to engage in spiritual-care interventions, such as meditation, that are not congruent with a patient's cultural values or religious beliefs (Cornette, 2005; Garces-Foley, 2006).

As found in studies on health-care providers (Daaleman et al., 2008; MacConville, 2006), a patient's spiritual and/or religious needs may not be addressed out of respect for patient privacy and autonomy; however, it could be that staff do not recognize or know how to handle spiritual and/or religious issues should they emerge. This could create a barrier to spiritual care that undermines a patient's life quality. As stated by a nurse in MacConville's (2006) study:

> If somebody has things that they need to get off their chest, if somebody has difficulty and wants to sort those out, and we offer that to them and they know that if you need us, we will be glad to help if you want us, I think they will take advantage of that opportunity if they want it. But I don't see the point in stirring things up and getting them more anxious at a point in their lives that they are just devastated on many fronts. . . . If we have any faith, if you do believe in a God then we say God is all-powerful, all-knowing, all-loving, well, if he or she is, then why not leave it up to God . . . why try to play God?
>
> (pp. 146–147)

This nurse did not seem to recognize that her personal feelings and beliefs could have influenced her receptivity to patient needs. Although a theistic perspective was assumed, the caregiver failed to acknowledge that the patient might have spiritual needs that were not articulated and thus could go unmet (Hermann, 2007). Hospice social workers must be aware that a patient may have spiritual needs and follow-up to ensure patient access to spiritual care.

PURPOSE OF SPIRITUAL CARE

Patients who are challenged by terminal illness may need assistance in finding strength, hope, meaning, comfort, and healing. This requires compassionate care in which one is fully present with the patient facing terminal illness (MacConville, 2006; Puchalski, 2001; Wright, 2002). Congruent with the purpose of hospice care, the purpose of spiritual care is to palliate, that is, "to soothe or relieve" suffering (Otis-Green, 2006, p. 1478). Spiritual care can be a proactive way to reduce and/or prevent spiritual suffering as well as to meet a patient's spiritual need for well-being (Peteet & Balboni, 2013; Stephenson et al., 2003; Swinton & Pattison, 2010). As described by Driscoll (2001), "Spiritual care discovers, reverences and tends the spirit—that is the energy, or the place of meaning and values—of another human being" (p. 2). Consistent with the idea of relational spirituality, the therapeutic relationship can enhance life meaning, as spiritual care is "relational and is given in relationship to others" (Edwards et al., 2010, p. 764; Murray et al., 2004; Smith, 2006). In the process, "spiritual care for hospice patients involves forging meaningful connections, respecting the patients' choices for managing their dying, and eliciting stories about life and death" (Stephenson et al., 2003, p. 51). This means spiritual care serves to build and/or sustain spiritual resilience. Spiritual care thus has the potential to soothe spiritual suffering and to promote spiritual well-being (Langegard & Ahlberg, 2009).

Swinton and Pattison (2010) describe spiritual care as an "activity" or "series of tasks" that support a patient's "quest" for spiritual well-being (p. 8). For example, a patient may feel life has little value. Spiritual care may involve affirming a patient's life experiences and helping a patient retain a sense of dignity as life comes to an end (Daaleman et al., 2008; Edwards et al., 2010). An interdisciplinary approach would be required to support life quality as the person nears death. This may include a need for community resources that involve a referral to a patient's personal spiritual-care provider. In a study of spiritual-care providers, Wright (2002) found that

> spiritual care affirms the value of each and every individual. It acknowledges the place of cultural traditions and personal relationships. It is based on empathy and non-judgemental love, affirming the worth of each person in the eyes of God. It responds to religious and non-religious spiritual needs by

meeting both the requirements of faith and the humanistic desire for another person to "be there," to listen, and to love . . . up to the point of death.

(p. 127)

Spiritual care begins with meeting people where they are and providing the type of care they are ready to receive (Chochinov & Cann, 2005; Daaleman et al., 2008; Puchalski, 2001; Wright, 2002). This involves being a companion and partnering with patients in the midst of illness and suffering (Puchalski, 2008b, 2008c; Puchalski et al., 2006). This also involves assisting patients either directly or indirectly to connect with what gives them meaning, hope, and strength (Chochinov & Cann, 2005; Edwards et al., 2010; Puchalski et al., 2006).

Edwards et al. (2010) systematically analyzed qualitative research on spiritual care at the end of life published between 2001 and 2009. Based on these data, relationships were central to the meaning-making process consistent with the idea of relational spirituality. Patients often expressed a desire to focus on experiencing a "spirit-to-spirit" relationship with others and a divine higher power as part of spiritual care (p. 753). For relationships with health-care providers to be therapeutic, an atmosphere of trust that was cultivated by a sharing of a common humanity through a willingness to be present, attentive, reflective, empathic, and respectful was required. Edwards et al. found that patients most closely identified with the relational aspects of palliative and hospice care. Through these relationships, patients satisfied their needs for involvement, optimism, control, closure, and normality. It seemed it was the experience of enhanced life meaning that made these relationships therapeutic. What detracted was an atmosphere of mistrust, evoked, for example, by feeling judged or being proselytized to by a palliative- or hospice-care provider. Therefore, the authors cautioned against focusing on spiritual care as a means of helping patients search for meaning without considering how relationships inform such meaning. Edwards et al. also stressed the importance of assuming responsibility for creating the conditions for a meaningful experience with patients.

Conclusion

A review of research to define spiritual care suggests that what defines spiritual care and who is considered to be a qualified spiritual-care provider has evolved over the years. Other professionals like nurses, social workers, and psychologists have joined chaplains in the provision of spiritual care. In the process, there has been a move away from a theistic approach, traditionally employed by chaplains, to a more humanistic approach, employed by other interdisciplinary team members. This has increased patient access to spiritual care, but it may lead to new problems associated with patient access to *quality* spiritual care. Spiritual care delivered by interdisciplinary team members allows for the integration of spiritual care throughout the provision of care, but the inclusion of spiritual care also demands a heightened awareness of a patient's spiritual needs, professional expertise, and interdisciplinary collaboration. Hospice social workers can draw from therapeutic qualities and skills to cultivate a spiritually sensitive relationship that is a spiritual resource for patients. This will likely involve continued education to build spiritual competence. However, some patients may still require spiritual care beyond the expertise of a hospice social worker that necessitates, for example, a referral to a chaplain with training to provide religious care. Therefore, an interdisciplinary approach is essential to ensuring patient access to quality spiritual care.

MODELS OF SPIRITUAL CARE

Diverse concepts, competencies, and strategies outlined in spiritual-care models can inform hospice social work (Glasper, 2011; Holloway et al., 2011). Based on a systematic review of research from 2000 to 2010 by Holloway et al. (2011), the authors found 12 spiritual-care models developed in various clinical settings only some of which were providing palliative and hospice care. They ranged from individual to organizational models and from theoretical to empirical models. The authors broadly categorized these models as conceptual, competency, whole-person synergy, interdisciplinary, and organizational. These models were not specifically designed for hospice social workers, but several will be reviewed to demonstrate how related principles may support the delivery of spiritually sensitive hospice social work. Two whole-person-synergy models will be explored with a reference to Sulmasy's (2002) biopsychosocial-spiritual model and Smith's (2006) synergy model. These models demonstrate how the delivery of spiritual care relies on the building of relationships that includes a respect for diversity, spiritual assessment, and continuing education. An interdisciplinary spiritual-care model will then be examined, given the importance of collaboration and referral in spiritually sensitive hospice social work. This interdisciplinary spiritual-care model was developed by Puchalski et al. (2009). The review ends with a description of how Callahan's (2013) relational model for spiritually sensitive hospice social work provides a foundation for spiritual care.

Whole-Person-Synergy Models

Whole-person-synergy spiritual-care models demonstrate how diverse and interacting factors make each person's experience of dying unique (Holloway et al., 2011). According to Sulmasy (2002), illness disrupts the relationships between the biopsychosocial and spiritual dimensions of a person inside and outside the body. As described by Sulmasy:

> Inside the body, the disturbances are twofold: (a) the relationships between and among the various body parts and biochemical processes, and (b) the relationship between the mind and the body. Outside the body, these disturbances are also twofold: (a) the relationship between the individual patient and his or her environment, including the ecological, physical, familial, social, and political nexus of relationships surrounding the patient; and (b) the relationship between the patient and the transcendent.
>
> (p. 26)

Even though these dimensions are connected, "each aspect can be affected differently by a person's history and illness, and each aspect can interact and affect other aspects of the person" (p. 27). The experience of dying can put intense strain on relationships. Intervention may be needed to help patients restore these relationships. According to Sulmasy:

> No matter what the patient's spiritual history, dying raises for the patient questions about the value and meaning of his or her life, suffering, and death. Questions of value are often subsumed under the term "dignity." Questions of meaning are often subsumed under the word "hope." Questions of relationship are often expressed in the need for "forgiveness." To die believing that one's life and death have been of no value is the ultimate indignity. To die believing that there is no meaning to life, suffering, or death is abject hopelessness. To die alone and unforgiven is utter alienation. For the

clinician to ignore these questions at the time of greatest intensity may be to abandon the patient in the hour of greatest need. So, the appropriate care of dying persons requires attention to the restoration of all the intrapersonal and extrapersonal relationships that can still be addressed, even when the patient is dying.

(p. 26)

A spiritual assessment can be used to explore the complex nature of these relationships and determine how to assist the patient in restoring "right relationships" for holistic healing. Sulmasy recognized that spirituality can be difficult to measure but may be understood based on quantifiable aspects of a patient's spirituality. These aspects include degree of patient's religiosity, spiritual/religious needs, spiritual/religious coping, and spiritual well-being.

Consistent with the whole-person approach, Smith's (2006) synergy model suggests the importance of addressing a patient's biopsychosocial and spiritual needs. Although this model was developed for nurses, it seems it could also inform hospice social workers, as it focuses on creating the conditions for a synergistic, helping relationship to emerge. Competency in caring practices and sensitivity to diversity are core components of this model that entails spiritual awareness and skill development to provide spiritual care. It is expected that hospice social workers would likewise need to cultivate caring connections marked by respect and "mutual knowing" as part of the healing environment (p. 44). This healing environment is said to allow for ongoing spiritual assessment. Spiritual assessment would help hospice social workers identify patient spiritual needs and access to spiritual resources. Spiritual intervention would likewise involve encouraging patients to draw from spiritual resources and practices that provide comfort. More utilization of spiritual resources is expected to increase the potential for a positive outcome, and so this model stresses resource availability and patient resiliency. External connections to additional resources may be needed to expand patient access. Also, based on this model, patients with particular characteristics or needs should be matched with hospice social workers with complementary expertise or competencies. This matching might not be possible beyond insuring a hospice social worker's level of spiritual competence is congruent with a patient's spiritual needs, which may necessitate a referral to a provider with more expertise.

Interdisciplinary Models

Interdisciplinary models demonstrate how hospice social workers may work with other professionals to facilitate the delivery of spiritual care (Holloway et al., 2011). As described in chapter 1, the National Consensus Project for Quality Palliative Care (NCP, 2015), founded in 2001, consists of experts across disciplines who have worked together to develop palliative-care guidelines in the United States. These guidelines include recommendations for eight domains of care with spiritual, religious, and existential aspects of care being among them (Dahlin, 2013; Puchalski, 2008c). As part of the NCP, Puchalski et al. (2009) developed an interdisciplinary model of spiritual care. They described this model as being relational as well as patient centered, since interdisciplinary team members and patients are required to engage in dialogue and collaborate throughout the delivery of care. This may involve shared decision making that extends to the patient's larger community of informal caregivers (Puchalski et al., 2006). They assert that all people who participate in coordinating spiritual care "have the potential for being transformed by interaction with one another," which suggests relational spirituality may be part of this experience (Puchalski et al., 2009, p. 890).

The provision of spiritual care begins with taking a spiritual history upon patient admission that includes an assessment of biopsychosocial issues to determine whether particular factors, including spiritual or religious beliefs, influence a patient's understanding of illness (Puchalski, 2008a, 2008b, 2008c). This further enables the development of a holistic approach to care "that honors the spiritual as well as the physical" (Puchalski, 2008b, p. 115). As this is generalist-specialist model of care, a BCC is considered to be a key resource in treatment planning and intervention, particularly when spiritual issues need to be addressed with a level of expertise beyond the competency or responsibility of interdisciplinary team members (Puchalski et al., 2006). This model focuses on creating the conditions for the delivery of compassionate care indicated by interdisciplinary team members who are "present to patients in the midst of their suffering and to work with patients out of a service-oriented, altruistic model of care" (Puchalski, 2008c, p. 38). An atmosphere of caring compassion is to be combined with the communication of genuine interest in the patient to help the patient feel comfortable in sharing spiritual concerns. This is what further supports the delivery of spiritual care as a patient-centered approach congruent with hospice social work.

More specifically, there are intrinsic and extrinsic components of care that are believed to be associated with the delivery of spiritual care. This begins to suggest the importance of drawing from therapeutic qualities and skills to engage in spiritual care, particularly when there is limited chaplain support (Peteet & Balboni, 2013). Extrinsic components of care involve the application of technical aspects, such as the ability to assess and address a patient's spiritual needs (Puchalski, 2008b; Puchalski et al., 2006). How these skills manifest may vary based on professional role, training, and context. As described by Puchalski et al. (2006):

> A physician may obtain data from a spiritual history, the nurse during bathing of the patient, and the social worker during a family conference. The chaplain, as the trained spiritual care professional works with the rest of the team by addressing the spiritual issues with patients more in-depth and assisting the rest of the team with creation and implementation of the spiritual treatment plan.
>
> (p. 414)

Intrinsic components of care are personal qualities internalized by the hospice social worker. These include attributes such as compassion, caring, intentionality, altruism, respect, openness, commitment, centeredness, and intuitiveness (Puchalski, 2008b; Puchalski et al., 2006). The model also suggests that hospice social workers need "to have a sense of who they are as spiritual beings—what gives their personal and professional lives meaning and purpose, how are they nurtured spiritually and how they find hope in the midst of caring for patients who are seriously ill and dying" (Puchalski et al., 2006, p. 414).

CENTRALITY OF RELATIONSHIP

These models suggest that the therapeutic relationship is central to the provision of spiritual care. Although there are many ways to understand spirituality, it is through relationships that patients may encounter the sacred. As described by Sandage and Shults (2007), "relating to the sacred" is what defines relational spirituality. Being in relationship with patients nearing the end of life allows hospice social workers to honor the sacredness of life and mysteries of death. However, even if "all spirituality can be viewed as relational (i.e., ways of relating to the sacred), not all forms of spirituality are relationally-constructive" (p. 263). How patients relate to the sacred through relationships might not always be positive. During periods of transition, like the dying process, spirituality can be marked by a loss of hope and spiritual suffering. Such experiences may be necessary and formative but do not immediately lend themselves to producing a positive spiritual state. The experience of spirituality may not always be positive, but this does not mean spiritual suffering leads to a permanent loss of vitality or fails to inform coping. Rather, there is a reciprocal relationship between spirituality and human development in which both positive and negative experiences of spirituality can be formative and lead to changes in relationships that may extend beyond a patient's life. Relating to that which is now and reaching for what could be creates a tension that must be balanced in the therapeutic relationship. For hospice social workers, this requires the ability to balance the discomfort of spiritual suffering with confidence in the power of spiritual resilience (Krieglstein, 2006).

A Relational Model

Multiple factors within the therapeutic relationship make the spiritual-care process complex. This reflects the importance of understanding what factors might directly and/or indirectly affect the therapeutic process (Chatters & Taylor, 2003). As noted in previous chapters, therapeutic qualities and skills of hospice social workers are important in providing spiritual care. Patients are believed to have their own experiences of spirituality, spiritual needs, and spiritual resources. Mobilizing spiritual resources to facilitate patient coping is believed to sustain and/or build spiritual resilience. One of these resources may be the therapeutic relationship. Hospice social workers have the capacity to honor a patient's need to feel spiritually supported within the limits of professional boundaries and level of spiritual competence. This enables a spiritually sensitive relationship that provides patients with a safe space for healing.

Extending the work of Canda and Furman (1999, 2010) and Faver (2004), Callahan (2009b, 2011b, 2012, 2013, 2015) suggested that spiritually sensitive hospice social work is a type of therapeutic relationship that validates the dignity and worth of a patient, congruent with social work professional ethics (NASW, 2008). Based on Buber's (1970) theory of dialogue, Callahan (2009) proposed that spiritual sensitivity requires an I-thou style of communication indicated by, for example, being authentic, responsive, and affirming. This review was followed by a qualitative study in which Callahan (2013) interviewed 16 nonpastoral hospice providers to learn how they provided spiritually sensitive care. As seen in figure 6.1, a relational model was developed that provides a foundation for spiritually sensitive hospice social work to be used as a form of spiritual care.

The model in figure 6.1 is based on the premise that the experience of relational depth is fluid, but spiritually sensitive hospice social work has the potential to be life transforming for both patient and hospice social worker. The experience of spiritual sensitivity is the result of an interaction of various factors, but the model focuses on the primary role of individual factors. Individual factors start with patient and hospice social worker readiness for the encounter. This would involve the patient's expression of spiritual needs and the hospice social worker's ability to engage in spiritual assessment. A referral would follow if patient needs extend beyond the scope of the hospice social worker's expertise. Subsequent intervention would entail the hospice social worker's application of therapeutic qualities and skills to engage in care provision that communicates spiritual sensitivity. These qualities and skills include being present, therapeutic touch,

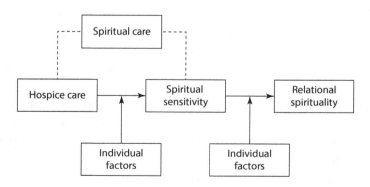

FIGURE 6.1 Relational model of spiritually sensitive hospice care.
Source: Callahan (2013).

recognizing personhood, listening, singing, reframing, affirming, self-disclosure, normalization, and advocacy with examples of each drawn from Callahan (2011, p. 24).

RECOGNIZING PERSONHOOD

In recognizing personhood, hospice providers said it was important to "see beyond" a patient's sickness and relate to the patient as a person. One hospice provider described it like this: "I was at a patient's house a few weeks ago. He did not have much to say . . . I saw a hiking stick in the corner. He said he and his wife both used to [go hiking. His wife said] he makes those hiking sticks . . . I started telling him I have a grandson who is starting to whittle. The patient just came alive." Another hospice provider said: "If you can just show a person that you care, that you are not afraid of what disease they have . . . I go in there and give them all the love I can . . . It doesn't matter what their religious denomination is or how their life may have been in the past."

THERAPEUTIC TOUCH/BEING PRESENT/LISTENING

Compassion was also communicated "without ever saying a word" by "the gentleness of the way you turn a patient" and when you "sit in silence with the patient." This was especially important when the patient was not alert or unresponsive. As described by one hospice provider: "A lot of these conversations are one or two words since people are going in and out of conscious[ness] with the disease process. They ask you not to leave. They fall asleep in the middle of telling you something and you move a little bit and they wake up and continue what they were saying."

BEING PRESENT/THERAPEUTIC TOUCH/SINGING

Spiritual care even included singing as demonstrated by this account:

> The more accepting . . . loving . . . and attentive I am, the more comfortable and open they become with me . . . One of my patients . . . loves hymns so I started singing to her. The next thing I know she is trying to sing with me. She is holding my hand and wants me to keep singing. I think touch is so important so I started to rub her head. She said to me when I was finished singing "Just sing one more song . . . just let's sing one more song."

RECOGNIZING PERSONHOOD/BEING PRESENT/THERAPEUTIC TOUCH

Over time, some hospice providers cultivated deep care for their patients as they began to relate to one another on a more personal level.

> Patients need a hospice worker who . . . is willing to let down their guard and show that they really care about them . . . If there is ever a time when people . . . need someone to care, it is when they are dying . . . I tell them that I will be looking forward to seeing them next time . . . I try to extend physical contact in some way that is not uncomfortable such as a casual patting [of] the arm and squeezing [of] the hand.

The second set of interventions associated with interpersonal support were said to be more clinical in nature, for they required advanced skills to communicate spiritual sensitivity. Clinical interventions included reframing, affirmation, self-disclosure, normalization, and advocacy.

REFRAMING

One hospice provider used reframing to help a patient gain new life meaning by challenging the patient to consider the impact of being a father. The hospice provider said:

> I worked with a man who was not religious . . . He said I have nothing. I said but you do have a daughter finishing high school about to go in to college. She wants to be a pediatrician. That may be your big purpose in your life. Maybe you were not there to help your daughter when she was young, but you still had an impact on her. The world is a different place because of you.

AFFIRMING/SELF-DISCLOSURE

Hospice providers tried to be universal in their approach, but also drew from specific knowledge of a patient's faith to meet the patient's spiritual needs. In one account, the hospice provider affirmed patient beliefs and engaged in self-disclosure to help the patient find comfort in their shared beliefs about an afterlife.

> I will use whatever . . . the patient brings up. I will affirm it . . . If they are people of Christian faith and they express their faith, I will affirm my

own Christian faith. I will join them as a believer by affirming them . . .
I try to reaffirm whatever their faith has taught them. I can reflect it back to
them by using the . . . words of their own church.

NORMALIZATION/ADVOCACY

In the next example, normalization was used to educate family members
about phenomena associated with the dying process and as a form of advocacy to ensure family members respected the patient's experience.

Many times patients will talk with family members who have already gone
on. I will tell those who are concerned about the patient's behavior that it is
very common . . . We don't know . . . Maybe the patients are talking to their
loved ones. If . . . they see things that we do not see. That does not make it
less real to them.

ADVOCACY

Patient advocacy further involved the solicitation of interpersonal support
for and on behalf of patients. This required awareness of the risk for neglect
of patient spiritual needs and potential for spiritual pain as seen in the following example:

It was right about the end of this patient's life . . . At that time, the daughter
was called in. She said "Daddy don't go." I just bluntly told her "Don't say
that to him. Don't you dare hold him back here like that." She then expressed
affirmation of his departure. He calmed right back down and passed . . . A
patient will be holding on for a long time until they get permission to go . . .
That spiritual support brings them peace.

Hospice providers consistently reflected a profound desire to reduce
patient spiritual pain. In the process, interpersonal support emerged as an
integral component of spiritual care. As one respondent expressed it, "We
only die once . . . I do believe it makes a difference."

Determining Success

The therapeutic effect of spiritually sensitive hospice social work is based on
the belief that there are times when the therapeutic relationship can be used

by a hospice social worker and be experienced by a patient as life enhancing. This reflects the value added in having a hospice social worker engage with the patient. Based on Callahan's (2013) qualitative study on hospice providers, relating seemed to have conveyed an interpersonal intimacy between hospice provider and patient during the provision of care that supported life meaning. It was this experience of enhanced life meaning or relational spirituality that indicated the style of hospice-care delivery was spiritually sensitive. For example, hospice providers consistently reported that they felt the primary purpose of their professional role was to facilitate patient comfort and connection. Hospice providers described being inspired. One hospice provider said "I take it to heart . . . This is where [God] uses me." Another said "[You] can feel God's presence" when providing spiritual care. This experience further inspired treatment innovation like a referral for spiritual care in an effort to relieve terminal agitation. Patient reactions to the provision of spiritual care suggested that the helping relationship was meaningful to them as well. Patients "expressed fulfillment" as they reached out to the hospice providers to "hug my neck" and say "thank you" and that "they love me." It appeared that both hospice providers and patients experienced relational spirituality.

Therefore, based on the work of Callahan, individual factors of both hospice provider and patient have the potential to influence the delivery of spiritually sensitive hospice social work. The experience of relational spirituality would be the anticipated result of spiritually sensitive hospice social work. Given the purpose of hospice social work is to support patients, the patient's perception of spiritual sensitivity is paramount, although a hospice social worker may also experience life enhancement through the process of providing spiritually sensitive care. It is also important to note that this model provides a useful guide for intervention but is limited in capturing the full scope of reality. For example, a significant limitation of Callahan's work is the focus on hospice providers. The experience of patients would need to be considered to determine what they perceive to be spiritually sensitive or how they might experience relational spirituality. Spiritually sensitive hospice social work necessitates ongoing collection of patient information that includes observing nonverbal cues in the process of delivering care. This feedback allows the hospice social worker to adjust the style of engagement to help the patient have a therapeutic, spiritually sensitive experience. Although hospice social workers should conduct spiritual assessments to help them learn more about the spiritual quality of care, authentic experience sometimes transcends what can be predicted or evaluated (Skovholt, 2005).

Congruence with Social Work

Although there are formal spiritual-care providers on interdisciplinary teams who are directly responsible for addressing the spiritual needs of patients, a patient's spiritual needs may also emerge in relationships with hospice social workers (Reese, 2013). Hospice social workers must be sensitive to a patient's spiritual needs and signs of spiritual suffering to be spiritually supportive. It is "communion with and service to other beings," Achterberg and Rothberg (1996) say, "[that] help us to get at aspects of our fear, grief, hatred, and ignorance, as well as our generosity, love, and insight, that are not necessarily accessible through individual spiritual practice" (p. 2). It requires a spiritual awareness or "staying awake to the sacred nature of relationships. . . . It's staying awake to the way that our everyday practice with others helps to bring consciousness to another level, helps us see each other more and more as sacred beings" (p. 5). It is through spiritually sensitive care that relationships provide a spiritual resource that enables the meeting of spiritual needs. In the process of engaging in spiritually sensitive care, hospice social workers may experience a heightened awareness of spirituality (Edwards et al., 2010; Puchalski et al., 2006; Stanworth, 2006). The profundity of such realizations may leave hospice social workers not knowing what to say to their patients as they face death other than simply being present with them. In this way, even silence provides a means of being spiritually sensitive as the hospice social worker stands as a witness to a patient's journey.

Therefore, a therapeutic relationship provides a way hospice social workers may engage in a form of spiritual care that has the potential to transform both patient and social worker. A relational approach to spiritually sensitive hospice social work is based on the idea that relationships enable patients to experience enhanced life meaning that builds and/or sustains spiritual resilience. Callahan's (2013) relational model provides a framework for intervention that may likewise be experienced by a patient as a form of spiritual care. Spiritually sensitive hospice social work is characterized by the intentional application of therapeutic qualities and skills congruent with traditional social work practice to enhance the *spiritual* quality of care. Social work values of service, social justice, dignity and worth of the person, importance of human relationships, integrity, and competence all support the sacredness of life (NASW, 2008). Likewise, patient self-determination, cultural competence, and respect for diversity are congruent with spiritually sensitive hospice social work (NASW, 2004, 2015). Building on the concept of relational spirituality, spiritually sensitive hospice social work may lead to the experience of enhanced life meaning that facilitates spiritual resilience. The process of engaging in spiritually sensitive hospice social work may further inspire hospice social workers to sustain care despite challenges that are inevitable in the practice of social work (Faver, 2004; Krieglstein, 2006; Seyfried, 2007). Spiritually sensitive hospice social work thus draws from the centrality of relationships in social work practice to honor the sacredness of a patient's life and death.

CONCLUSION

Hospice social workers are among key professionals hospice patients will encounter as they near the end of life and must be equipped to respond to myriad needs. To support the delivery of quality hospice care, hospice social workers must maximize opportunities to enhance the spiritual quality of care (NCP, 2013; NQF, 2006). This is particularly important when patients present with spiritual needs that require immediate intervention (Reese, 2013). Whole-person-synergy models suggest that the cultivation of helping relationships requires respect for diversity, spiritual assessment, and continuing education (Smith, 2006; Sulmasy, 2002). Interdisciplinary models of spiritual care stress the importance of collaboration and referral with BCCs to provide a resource for specialized intervention (Puchalski et al., 2009). Callahan's (2013) relational model provides a foundation for spiritual care in which hospice social workers cultivate a therapeutic relationship that has the potential to help patients experience enhanced life meaning. This approach is congruent with traditional social work practice but requires intentional application. Additional model testing is needed to explore the potential for factors to interact in the process of providing spiritually sensitive hospice social work; some of these factors may not be controlled through skilled intervention. Toward this end, the next chapter will focus on the delivery of spiritually sensitive hospice social work.

7

Spiritual Sensitivity

PALLIATIVE- AND HOSPICE-CARE RESEARCH HAS increasingly focused on patient spirituality with evidence to suggest spiritual support enhances quality of life (Balboni et al., 2007; Sinclair et al., 2006). It is important to know what kind of spiritual support, if any, patients want from hospice social workers. Spiritually sensitive hospice social work enables hospice social workers to recognize a patient's spiritual needs and signs of spiritual suffering, including what patients want for spiritual care. The process of being spiritually sensitive does not mean a social worker must engage in the delivery of spiritual care. Spiritual care may not directly involve hospice social workers, but spiritually sensitive hospice social work does provide an appropriate way to respond. Patients may simply want hospice social workers to have meaningful relationships with them (Edwards et al., 2010). Hospice social workers can draw from particular qualities and skills to cultivate the spiritual quality of care that has the potential to enhance life meaning (Callahan, 2009a, 2013). This chapter will clarify how to engage in spiritually sensitive hospice social work, starting with clarifying what it means to be spiritually sensitive.

BEING SENSITIVE TO PATIENT NEEDS

Throughout the phases of terminal illness, patients may experience spiritual needs as well as the potential for spiritual suffering. They may need spiritual support, but research remains unclear about how patients want hospice providers to respond, with even less information available specific to hospice social workers (Taylor & Mamier, 2004). There are some patients who have expressed a desire for hospice providers to be responsive to their spiritual needs. For example, patients may want someone to discuss their doubts about life after death but fear being rejected by their religious community if they are perceived as questioning their faith (Puchalski, 2008a). Patients may not be religious but still want to have meaningful relationships with hospice providers in a positive, caring environment (Chochinov & Cann, 2005; Edwards et al., 2010; Nixon & Narayanasamy, 2010; Sulmasy, 2009; Taylor & Mamier, 2004). Patients may want spiritual needs to inform hospice care, which may include praying together (Chochinov & Cann, 2005; Puchalski, 2008b; Sulmasy, 2009). Other patients may not want to express spiritual concerns, particularly when hospice providers have limited time for support, patients fear distracting hospice providers from delivering primary care, think hospice providers might not understand them, or lack the professional expertise to help (Chochinov & Cann, 2005; Hills et al., 2005; Nixon & Narayanasamy, 2010; Pesut, 2008b). Patients may want to avoid hospice providers whom they fear would give spiritual advice or "preach" to them (Edwards et al., 2010). Given so many concerns, it is hard to know what patients would consider is spiritually sensitive.

Taylor and Mamier (2004) conducted a mixed-methods study using a convenience sample of 156 patients and 68 family caregivers to determine what kind of spiritual support patients wanted from nurses. The authors observed that patients varied widely in their expectations. Patients were most enthusiastic about being able to address their own spiritual needs, rather than being subject to more intrusive and hierarchical methods. In order of preference, patients wanted spiritual care that involved the use of humor, to be given assistance in having personal space or quiet time, and for nurses to pray for them. They were least likely to want to be taught how to draw or write about their spirituality or discuss their difficulties in praying while sick. Similarly, Hermann (2007) suggested that when patients could meet their own spiritual needs, those needs were met at a higher rate than when patients required the assistance of others. Taylor and Mamier (2004) further noted that patient religiosity seemed to have some influence over a desire for spiritual care. There were also patients who considered spirituality a private matter, had other people to share their spiritual concerns with, or did not want to discuss their spiritual concerns with a nurse they did not know well. The authors warned against making assumptions about patient wishes and recommended conducting a spiritual assessment to inform care.

However, these findings also suggested the need to consider whether pictorial assessments, such as a spiritual life map used to illustrate a patient's spiritual history, would be appropriate (Hodge, 2003, 2005b). It is unknown whether patients would have felt the same way about hospice social workers, but perhaps so, given that spiritual care extends outside the boundaries of traditional social work practice and nursing care alike.

Sloan et al. (2000) questioned physicians who address religious issues with patients. Their comments would also apply to hospice social workers, since religious care requires a referral to a formal spiritual-care provider. Sloan et al. suggested that providing religious care as a form of spiritual care raised ethical questions and threatened patient autonomy. The authors contended that even if patients wanted physicians to address religious issues, this did not make it appropriate to do so. Under different circumstances, physicians would not encourage patients to get married or have children to gain the positive health benefits of such choices. These choices, like religion, are personal choices. Furthermore, physicians risked patient coercion, given their position of authority. The provision of religious care could lead to an attribution of professional expertise beyond that of physicians. Treating religious practices like any other psychosocial intervention further risked oversimplifying any potential connection with a therapeutic outcome. For example, counting how often a patient prayed could fail to accurately reflect the qualitative benefits of prayer. As stated by Sloan et al., "Religion is more than a collection of views and practices, and its value cannot be determined instrumentally; it is a spiritual way of being in the world" (p. 1916). Thus, addressing religious issues without training could risk trivializing them. Pesut (2008b) echoed this concern by saying "at a time when I might need a supportive spiritual presence more than any other time in my life, I would be confronted by a professional discourse that trivializes my reality, and worse, dismisses it as untrue" (p. 136).

Considering the risk for patients to experience spiritual harm, variability in their desire for spiritual support is understandable. It can also be hard to determine how best to spiritually support these patients. Palliative- and hospice-care research on spirituality has been growing, but studies have failed to be conclusive in defining best practices, as they are few in number and have conceptual and measurement issues and limited samples (Draper, 2011; Edwards et al., 2010; Gijsberts et al., 2011; Hodge & McGrew, 2005; McSherry et al., 2004; Okon, 2005; Pesut, Sinclair, Fitchett, Greig, & Koss,

2016; Pike, 2011; Sinclair et. al., 2006; Swinton & Pattison, 2010). Furthermore, there is a dearth of research on spiritual care delivered by hospice social workers, so it is unclear the extent to which research from other disciplines would apply to social work practice. Some researchers suggest that hospice social workers provide minimal support and are not comfortable addressing spiritual issues (Clausen et al., 2005; Puchalski et al., 2006; Stirling, 2007). Nevertheless, as described in chapter 1, social work leaders have clarified practice guidelines and provided training opportunities. Spiritual care may only require spiritual assessment and referral, but any provision of spiritual care assumes patients want hospice social workers to help. This may or may not be true. Spiritual sensitivity can help hospice social workers determine what kind of spiritual support patients prefer. Spiritual sensitivity further enables hospice social workers to coordinate with interdisciplinary team members to ensure continued access to spiritual care.

DEFINING SPIRITUAL SENSITIVITY

In social work and related fields, scholars have described the concept of spiritual sensitivity and how spiritual sensitivity may be expressed by helping professionals (Briggs & Rayle, 2005; Butot, 2005; Canda, 1999; Canda & Furman, 1999, 2010; Gause & Coholic, 2007; Krieglstein, 2006; Rice & McAuliffe, 2009; Sperry, 2010; Sperry & Miller, 2010). Canda and Furman (1999) defined spiritual sensitivity in social work practice as "a way of being and relating throughout the entire helping process" that provides a foundation for good social work practice (p. 186). As described by Canda and Furman (1999):

> All forms and types of social work activities can be consistent with spiritually sensitive practice when they are conducted within the framework of spiritually sensitive values and contexts for helping. Everything that furthers the spiritual fulfillment of people, individually and collectively, is spiritually sensitive when the practitioner is aware of and intentional about this.... This does not require that the practitioner speak explicitly about this with clients; this decision should be based on the best interests of clients. But it does require a spiritual vision of human capacity and possibility. This vision helps us to breathe new life (literally, "to inspire") into all our social activities.
>
> (pp. 282–283)

Canda (1999) suggests spiritual sensitivity inspires unconditional love, compassion, and a genuine desire to help patients. Social workers should treat patients as "full and complete persons, with inherent worthiness of respect . . . rather than diagnostic categories or bundles of problems or dysfunctions" (p. 9). Butot (2005) describes this type of approach as being spiritually informed. Spiritually informed practice assumes everything is interconnected and everyone is intrinsically valuable. Healing and change starts from this place of being a whole person rather than one who is broken in need of intervention. This "love in practice" is a way of perceiving, rather than a way of being or doing (n.p.).

There are therapeutic qualities and skills that are believed to reflect spiritual sensitivity. According to Butot (2005), social workers need the ability to attend, support, and offer tools or new ways of perceiving their circumstances. This process should involve responding to what is called the "compassionate challenge" to accept "not-knowing" and "what is," particularly when it is impossible to know what is best for others or advocating for a particular outcome would undermine patient autonomy. Canda and Furman (1999, 2010) detail other qualities that are required to be spiritually sensitive. Spiritually sensitive social workers must be able to communicate value clarity, respect, client centeredness, inclusivity, and creativity.

Value Clarity

A spiritually sensitive social worker needs to be clear about personal opinions and beliefs, particularly those from a spiritual and religious perspective. The implications of personal values need to be considered as they relate to professional values and service delivery. Practice guidelines set forth by the NASW provide a reference. Self-reflection that clarifies values and limitations of such also requires openness to growth. This open posture allows social workers to be more receptive to and encouraging of patients' expression of their unique spiritual views and beliefs.

Respect

A spiritually sensitive social worker must retain unconditional positive regard for patients and recognize that each person has inherent dignity and worth rather than engage in the process of objectifying or stereotyping the person. This entails cultivating Martin Buber's (1970) I-Thou relationship, in which the essence of a patient is valued and is authentically engaged as part of the therapeutic process. This process becomes an opportunity for the social worker to connect with the divine in each patient as the therapeutic encounter transforms into a spiritual encounter. Respect allows for receptivity to the mystery and possibility of each encounter.

Client Centeredness

A spiritually sensitive social worker is willing to understand a patient's worldview. This includes respect for patient spiritual beliefs and practices that are associated with a patient's worldview. Humility is required for social workers to recognize that they are not experts on what patients should do but rather are companions in the process of helping patients seek direction and find their own truths. Even when this process entails a responsibility to therapeutically intervene, such an approach is tempered by understanding, validation, and respect for the patient's experience to convey the social worker's underlying spirit of good will.

Inclusivity

A spiritually sensitive social worker is not only tolerant but is also affirming and inclusive of diversity among patients. This includes recognition of various spiritual beliefs and practices.

To exercise religious freedom and spiritual self-determination, advocacy might be required for patients who need additional spiritual resources. Social workers may need to engage in social networking, coordination of services, and continuing education that enhance their own understanding of spiritual and religious diversity.

Creativity

A spiritually sensitive social worker helps patients recognize the myriad possibilities in responding to life challenges. Beyond the experience of human suffering, patients also have the capacity for resilience nurtured by creative energies for self-transformation. Spiritually oriented activities may be a part of this process. For example, the creation of art may tap into aesthetic pleasures not accessible otherwise. This requires social workers to be flexible, spontaneous, and present in the moment to identify what inspires patient creativity. Social workers may need to directly help patients engage in this process for therapeutic ends to be realized.

Briggs and Rayle (2005) described spiritual sensitivity for professional counselors. These qualities are a natural extension of those suggested by Canda and Furman (1999, 2010) and thus provide another means of expressing spiritual sensitivity through counseling and other practice roles employed by social workers. Spiritual sensitivity is described as a genuine encounter between two people, the patient and counselor in this case, on a journey that involves the seeking of personal transformation through a therapeutic relationship. A spiritually sensitive counselor is said to cultivate a therapeutic relationship that reflects benevolent connectedness, unconditional and hopeful openness, and transcendent meaningfulness.

Benevolent Connectedness

A spiritually sensitive counselor approaches the therapeutic relationship as a partnership that is accepting of the patient and promotes healing. The emotional body is central to this partnership, but there is also a spiritual quality that is communicated through a felt experience of interconnectedness, even if this quality is not explicitly discussed. Therefore, the counselor seeks to affirm patient spirituality as this experience emerges from connections with self, others, and the counselor. This enables the therapeutic relationship to become a sacred relationship.

Unconditional and Hopeful Openness

A spiritually sensitive counselor is optimistic about the possibility of transformation through the therapeutic relationship. A spiritually sensitive counselor may directly or indirectly encourage hope in patients. Yalom (1995) described this process as the instillation of hope, which is considered a key therapeutic or curative factor. There is a shared commitment to joining in the difficult work of meaning making that may be required as part of this process. It is the hope and trust in the fruitfulness of the therapeutic work that helps make transformation possible.

Transcendent Meaningfulness

A spiritually sensitive counselor creates a therapeutic relationship that inspires the experience of meaning. Although a therapeutic relationship is challenging, therapeutic challenges occur in the context of an accepting relationship that inspires patient self-worth. A spiritually sensitive counselor communicates, for example, unconditional positive regard, empathy, and genuineness. This style of relating validates a patient's significance and can help patients transcend feelings of meaninglessness in the world.

Spiritual sensitivity enables social workers to operate from an open spiritual stance that communicates respect for patients and what makes their lives meaningful (Meador, 2006). This includes a genuine interest in helping patients clarify their values and beliefs without fear of judgment or pressure to change them (Briggs & Rayle, 2005). Proselytizing would be incongruent with creating a safe spiritual space, but other spiritually oriented activities might be in order. Canda and Furman (1999) provided a list of spiritually oriented activities, some of which are listed in box 7.1. The authors divided these activities into those that may be used with and by individuals, families, and groups and those that may be used with and by organizations and communities. These activities suggest social workers may engage in practices that are considered spiritually sensitive across systemic levels based on education and expertise (Briggs & Rayle, 2005; Canda & Furman, 1999; 2010).

SPIRITUALLY SENSITIVE HOSPICE SOCIAL WORK

According to Okon (2005), death is not a problem to be solved but a state of transformation that is shared within a narrative dwelling place. Hospice social workers can cultivate a therapeutic relationship for this narrative dwelling place. Spiritually sensitive hospice social workers have the capacity to support a patient's personhood by responding to a patient's spiritual need to be seen and validated as a person of dignity and worth. Spiritually sensitive hospice social workers can further mobilize spiritual resources. Some resources must be newly created to help patients build and/or sustain spiritual resilience. Such interventions require a hospice social worker to engage in ongoing spiritual assessment to understand a patient's spiritual needs and spiritual resources. Hence, a spiritually sensitive hospice social

BOX 7.1 EXAMPLES OF SPIRITUALLY ORIENTED HELPING ACTIVITIES

Practice with and by Individuals, Families, and Groups

1. Art, music, dance, poetry therapies
2. Assessing spiritual emergencies
3. Assessing spiritual propensity
4. Caring for the body
5. Cooperation with clergy, religious communities, and spiritual support groups
6. Cooperation with traditional healers
7. Creating a spiritual development timeline and narrative
8. Developing or participating in rituals and ceremonies
9. Dialoguing across spiritual perspectives
10. Differentiating between spiritual emergencies and psychopathology
11. Distinguishing between religious visions and hallucinations or delusions
12. Dream interpretation
13. Exploring family patterns and meaning and ritual
14. Exploring sacred stories, symbols, and teachings
15. Focused relaxing
16. Forgiveness
17. Guided visualization
18. Intentional breathing
19. Journaling and diary keeping
20. Meditation and prayer
21. Mindfulness
22. Nature retreats
23. Reading scripture and inspirational materials
24. Reflecting on policy regarding death and the afterlife
25. Reflecting on helpful or harmful impact of religious participation

Practice with and by Organizations and Communities

1. Advocacy for spiritual sensitivity in health and social service policy
2. Creating a spiritually sensitive administrative approach
3. Cooperation with clergy, religious communities, and spiritual support groups
4. Cooperation with traditional healers
5. Dialoguing across spiritual perspectives
6. Developing or participating in rituals and ceremonies
7. Exploring sacred stories, symbols, and teaching of spiritual communities

Source: Canda & Furman, 1999, pp. 291–292.

worker must balance being a learner and being a facilitator to enhance the spiritual quality of care (Briggs & Rayle, 2005; Canda & Furman, 1999; 2010). Callahan's (2009b, 2013, 2015) relational model provides a way for hospice social workers to apply the concept of spiritual sensitivity.

Callahan's (2009b, 2013, 2015) relational model for spiritually sensitive hospice social work provides a conceptual framework for the delivery of therapeutic interventions throughout the provision of care. Extending the work of Canda and Furman (1999, 2010), Callahan's model for spiritually sensitive hospice social work may likewise serve as a form of spiritual care. Spiritually sensitive hospice social work is a therapeutic style of engagement that can enhance a patient's life quality and can, thus, be experienced as meaningful. This experience of enhanced life meaning defines relational spirituality. When spiritually sensitive hospice social work indirectly meets a patient's spiritual needs, then it may be considered an implicit form of spiritual care. Spiritually sensitive hospice social work may also be used directly to meet a patient's spiritual needs as an explicit form of spiritual care, given the level of expertise of the hospice social worker. As such, traditional social work skills may be used for the delivery of implicit and explicit spiritual care.

Implicit Spiritual Care

Implicit interventions that indirectly address a patient's spiritual needs involve the application of generalist qualities and skills that define spiritual sensitivity (Callahan, 2015; Puchalski et al., 2009). Given the centrality of the therapeutic relationship, these generalist social work skills would seamlessly integrate into the delivery of spiritually sensitive hospice social work (Briggs & Rayle, 2005; Callahan, 2009a, 2012, 2013; Canda, 1999, 2005; Canda & Furman, 1999, 2010; Yardley, Walshe, & Parr, 2009). These skills provide an informal approach to spiritual care, as they nurture the spiritual quality of the therapeutic relationship, which includes professional boundaries to help hospice social workers remain in touch with professional roles and responsibilities. As described by Puchalski (2006):

> Compassionate care involves the caregiver's ability to share the patient's pain and suffering without becoming overwhelmed and disabled by that suffering. This love stems from an intimacy in which boundaries are respected for

both the patient and the caregiver—an intimacy with formality. The caregiver feels that pain and suffering of the other by being empathic, is able to help the other by understanding this suffering at an intuitive and felt level, but then is able to detach enough to be able to help guide the patient toward a self-healing of that suffering.

(p. 42)

Examples of generalist skills are listed in box 7.2 . This includes the ability to communicate compassion, empathy, respect, and being fully present, all of which may be applied in combination to validate the dignity and worth of a patient, congruent with social work professional ethics (NASW, 2008). Social workers are also likely to require the skills to engage in the roles of educator, advocate, mediator, and broker to facilitate access to formal spiritual care, for example, through a referral to a hospice chaplain (Callahan, 2015). Although these interventions are part of traditional social work, in spiritually sensitive hospice social work they may be used indirectly to provide spiritual care. As with any social work intervention, spiritually sensitive hospice social work requires the application of skills that are congruent with patient needs and are in line with professional boundaries relative to education and expertise.

Explicit Spiritual Care

Explicit interventions that directly address spiritual needs involve spiritually oriented activities, previously described as spiritual resources. This provides a formal means of spiritual care, although it is not intended to replace the services of a chaplain and/or other professional if patient needs exceed professional competence. Explicit spiritual-care interventions are expected to build upon generalist skills and interventions. Given the need for a more advanced skill set, the application of spiritually oriented activities as part of explicit spiritual care requires advanced generalist and/or clinical social work skills. Some of these spiritually oriented activities, which are drawn from hospice literature, are listed in box 7.1. These activities may involve patients engaging in prayer, meditation, or contemplation; enlisting the prayers of others; reading inspirational materials; and listening to spiritual music. They may also incorporate reliance on symbolism, imagery, or rituals/activities; positive affirmation; spiritual conversation; cultivating environmental and familial

BOX 7.2   EXAMPLES OF SPIRITUAL-CARE INTERVENTIONS

Generalist Interventions

Modes of delivery: therapeutic relationship, psycho-education, and supportive counseling (individual, family, and group).

1. Being compassionate
2. Being empathic/relating/understanding
3. Evidencing trustworthiness
4. Being affirming/valuing/respecting patient dignity/supporting/accepting/positive regard/humanizing/validating
5. Being kind/gentle/comforting/loving/nurturing/caring/warm/attending
6. Being a companion/patient-centered/providing personalized support/recognizing uniqueness/collaborative
7. Facilitating relationships
8. Focusing on the ordinariness of life
9. Maintaining good rapport/asking open questions/communicating skillfully
10. Expressing a genuine desire to understand/enjoying time together
11. Being present or available/connecting/offering a therapeutic touch/promising nonabandonment/being a witness to the patient's experience/accompanying the patient on this journey
12. Active listening/using silence effectively
13. Having self-awareness and spiritual knowing
14. Making a referral

Advanced Generalist/Clinical Interventions

Modes of delivery: therapeutic relationship, psycho-education, psychotherapy (individual, family, and group), and alternative.*

1. Completing a spiritual assessment
2. Facilitating spiritual expression/spiritual conversations
3. Setting flexible boundaries/offering reciprocal sharing
4. Providing guidance/problem solving
5. Enabling spiritual self-care/identifying inner resources/supporting personal belief systems
6. Identifying potential spiritual/religious resources
7. Offering bereavement counseling/end-of-life planning

BOX 7.2 (CONTINUED)

8. Aiding in life review/listening to reminiscences/enabling meaning making/ identifying ways to make memories

9. Inspiring hope

10. Reframing

11. Using humor

*Alternative modes of delivery include art therapy, music therapy, dream work, acupuncture, therapeutic touch, biofeedback, relaxation response, guided imagery, and aromatherapy.

Sources: Byock, 1996; Carroll, 2001; Cavendish et al., 2003; Chaturvedi, 2007; Chochinov & Cann, 2005; Cornette, 2005; Edwards et al., 2010; Exline et al., 2013; Ferrell, 2011; Glasper, 2011; Heyse-Moore, 1996; Hills et al., 2005; HPNA, 2013; Kisvetrova, Kluger, & Kabelka, 2013; Mako et al., 2006; Milligan, 2011; Mitchell et al., 2006; Narayanasamy, 2007; NHPCO, 2007; Okon, 2005; Penman et al., 2007; Puchalski, 2008a, 2008b, 2008c, 2013; Puchalski et al., 2006, 2009; Sperry, 2010; Sperry & Miller, 2010; Stern & James, 2006.

spiritual support; and identifying new spiritual resources. Explicit spiritual care includes spiritual assessment, the point at which intervention begins and is necessary to guide further intervention. There are clinical interventions that are designed specifically to help patients retain a sense of dignity and engage in meaning making, but details for application with hospice patients needs further research (Callahan, 2015; Chochinov & Cann, 2005; Okon, 2005).

Application of Interventions

Based on the work of Knight and von Gunten (2004b), box 7.3 illustrates how hospice social workers may apply generalist and advanced generalist/ clinical interventions to address specific spiritual needs of patients. Generalist skills may be used in the process of communicating compassion, empathy, respect, and kindness to respond to the spiritual need for patients to maintain a sense of self-worth. This could involve talking to patients rather than talking about patients while in their presence, even if patients are unable to completely understand what is being said. Hospice social workers may further engage patients as people first by sharing information, soliciting feedback, and using active listening to convey understanding of patient concerns. This may include exploring what helps the patient feel like a human being

BOX 7.3   EXAMPLES OF APPLYING SPIRITUAL-CARE INTERVENTIONS

Generalist Interventions

1. For the spiritual need to *maintain sense of self-worth*:
   a. Talk to patients rather than about patients in their presence, even if they are not clearly capable of complete understanding.
   b. Ask patients how they are doing or feeling before focusing on completing tasks.
   c. Engage patients in collaborative processes through information sharing and soliciting feedback in making choices.

2. For the spiritual need to *feel connected to the social world*:
   a. Ask patients to identify meaningful connections (such as with family, friends, workplace, school, civic groups, and religious/spiritual community).
   b. Encourage and facilitate ongoing involvement to maintain connections.
   c. If practical, help patients maintain a connection with their loved pets.

3. For the spiritual need to *overcome fears*:
   a. Encourage patients to talk about the sources of their fears.
   b. Actively listen to and acknowledge patient fears.
   c. Ask patients to describe sources of comfort or what provides a sense of order. This may include other people, spiritual and religious faith, and religious/spiritual rituals, including ordinary routine (e.g., bathing, preparing for bed).

Advanced Generalist/Clinical Interventions

1. For the spiritual need to *retain hope*:
   a. Normalize a patient's wish for death.
   b. Confirm that a patient is indeed growing weaker or has multiple symptoms that indicate death is near.
   c. Affirm that the patient's state will not go on forever.
   d. Ensure patients and families feel heard.

2. For the spiritual need to *resolve bitter feelings*:
   a. If the patient is upset over changing roles, help him or her consider what the changing role means, mourn losses, redefine, and affirm the new role.

BOX 7.3 *(CONTINUED)*

  b. If patients blame themselves or God, normalize feelings and engage in life review to provide some release from blame, even if suffering cannot be explained.
  c. Process anger with patients and help patients identify areas where they can facilitate conflict resolution and seek (self-)forgiveness.
  d. Refer to a chaplain or other formal spiritual-care provider if anger at God persists.

3. For the spiritual need to *gain closure*:
  a. Help patient, family, and friends cope with anticipatory grief.
  b. Encourage patient empowerment by helping patients identify areas where they can have input and exercise choice.
  c. Process negative feelings about the past with patients and help patients identify areas where they can facilitate conflict resolution and seek (self-) forgiveness.
  d. Ask interdisciplinary team members to help patients see the value in life accomplishments and take advantage of opportunities to finish business.

Adapted from: Knight and von Gunten, C. (2004b).

rather than just a "case" or a "patient." Advanced generalist/clinical interventions may be needed to directly address the spiritual need of patients to resolve bitter feelings. To express self-blame, patients might say, "I must have done something to deserve this kind of life." A hospice social worker could use clinical skills, such as normalization and reframing, as well as life review and conflict resolution, to help patients gain a sense of peace. Patients might blame God, leading to a need to talk to someone about religious issues, which would require a referral to a formal spiritual-care provider.

Depending on the skills necessary to help patients meet their spiritual needs, hospice social workers may use generalist, advanced generalist, and/or clinical interventions. This requires intentional efforts to engage in spiritually sensitive hospice social work and continuing education to help build spiritual competence. If a hospice social worker does not have the training to use advanced generalist and/or clinical interventions for explicit spiritual care, then consultation with interdisciplinary team members with more expertise, including the social worker's supervisor, is required. When spiritual needs require more than advanced generalist and/or clinical intervention, such as to resolve religious conflicts, the hospice social worker should ask whether the patient is willing to meet with a formal spiritual-care provider such as a hospice chaplain or religious/spiritual community leader. In any case, the practice of spiritually sensitive hospice social work to help patients meet their spiritual needs requires collaboration with interdisciplinary team members. Interdisciplinary team members can support the delivery of spiritual care provided they understand how the hospice social worker is trying to spiritually support patients. Collaboration can also ensure spiritual care is being delivered in a manner that is supportive of patients rather than causing patients to be confused about the involvement of different hospice professionals who may have conflicting approaches to the provision of spiritual care.

Spiritually sensitive hospice social work has been described as a dynamic process that involves the cultivation of a meaningful therapeutic relationship that is experienced as relational spirituality. This chapter reviewed therapeutic qualities and skills that provide the foundation for a spiritually sensitive intervention; however, being spiritually sensitive also depends on what a patient needs and experiences as being spiritually sensitive. This makes prescribed steps to provide spiritual care more difficult, if not misleading. Definitional boundaries risk distorting what might be experienced as spiritually sensitive given spiritual diversity. Hospice social workers must be able to tolerate some degree of ambiguity in what defines spiritual sensitivity. In addition, contrary to Smith's (2006) synergy model, spiritually sensitive hospice social work is not a product of practice techniques. Greater utilization of spiritual resources may not necessarily increase the potential for a positive outcome. For practical purposes, guidance is necessary for application, but ideally the hospice social worker should be able to draw from research, including practice wisdom and ethical/theoretical guidelines, to be *spiritually* sensitive to changing conditions. A level of spiritual sensitivity is needed to clarify which interventions support a patient's worldview and associated spiritual competence. Spiritually sensitive hospice social work thus assumes a foundation in social work education. One area that necessitates training is how to conduct a formal spiritual assessment, such as a spiritual history.

SPIRITUAL ASSESSMENT

When spiritually sensitive hospice social work is used to provide spiritual care, a spiritual assessment is necessary. The level of formality may vary based on a patient's needs, but the manner in which a spiritual assessment is conducted can be therapeutic (Okon, 2005). The conduct of a formal spiritual assessment as a therapeutic intervention requires training. This is why a spiritual assessment is considered an advanced generalist intervention. There are particular times when a formal spiritual assessment may be necessary (see table 7.1). For example, as described by Knight and von Gunten (2004c), spiritual needs and signs of spiritual suffering require further assessment:

> Health care providers may observe that a patient is very anxious or fearful or may hear statements suggesting the existence of despair or self-blame such as, "I must have done something wrong to deserve this kind of suffering." The patients may not consider themselves as very "spiritual" and therefore may decline a visit from the "chaplain." However, these kinds of issues are rightly included as part of the spiritual assessment.
>
> (n.p.)

Hospice social workers will need to be intentional about creating a spiritually sensitive environment that supports patient self-disclosure. Knight and von Gunten (2004a) caution that patients may express initial resistance, particularly if a patient has a history of spiritual abuse or religious discrimination. The patient may fear the hospice social worker might question the legitimacy of his or her religious beliefs. Social workers can, for example, draw from generalist interventions such as active listening, being present, and expressing positive regard.

Hospice social workers may encourage patients to share their spiritual concerns by simply asking if they have any (Milligan, 2011). To begin a formal spiritual assessment, it would be appropriate to tell patients why a spiritual assessment is needed. It may help to explain that information from the spiritual assessment will help the hospice social worker identify the most appropriate forms of care. It is also important to communicate respect for a patient's right to privacy and option to refuse a spiritual assessment (Edwards et al., 2010; Knight & von Gunten, 2004c; Meador,

TABLE 7.1 Reasons to Address Spirituality

TYPE	EXPLANATION
Patient expectations	Patient expresses a spiritual and/or religious worldview, reports a religious affiliation, and solicits spiritual support.
Spiritual needs	Patient relies on spiritual resources, expresses a desire for spiritual resources (has limited access to spiritual support), and reflects signs of spiritual suffering.
Developmentally appropriate	The dying process is considered a developmental stage of life with associated needs, such as the need to process emotional response to loss.
Change in medical status	First diagnosis, symptoms (remission/active dying), medication side effects, and duration (acute/chronic)
Component of holistic care	The tradition of hospice is to provide biopsychosocial-spiritual care that supports the collective needs of patients and their caregivers.
Mandated by accrediting organizations	The Joint Commission authorizes hospice providers for Medicare reimbursement.
Supported by professional organizations	Professional organizations across disciplines have recognized the importance of respect for patient spirituality. This includes social work organizations such as the National Association of Social Workers (NASW), Council on Social Work Education (CSWE), Society for Spirituality and Social Work (SSSW), and the North American Association of Christians in Social Work (NACSW).
Therapeutic effects	Spiritual resources, such as positive religious coping by maintaining faith through prayer and reconciliation, have the potential to enhance life quality.

Sources: Callahan, 2008, 2009a, 2009b, 2016; Canda & Furman, 1999, 2010; Carson & Koenig, 2004; CSWE, 2008, 2015a, 2015b, 2015c; Cunningham, 2012; Derezotes, 2006; Hermann, 2007; Hodge, 2003; Hodge & Bushfield, 2006; Horton-Parker & Fawcett, 2010; Joint Commission, 2016; Knight & von Gunten, 2004c; Koenig, 2007, 2008; Lee et al., 2009; Mathews, 2009; Mitchell et al., 2006; Murray et al., 2004; Murray et al., 2007; NACSW, 2008; NASW 2001, 2004, 2008, 2015; Pargament, 2007; Puchalski, 2006; Reese, 2013; SSSW, n.d.; Taylor, 2007.

2006; Mitchell et al., 2006; Okon, 2005). A patient's physical condition may also limit participation, and thus requires, for example, shorter periods of assessment time or the assistance of a caregiver with whom a patient is comfortable. In asking questions, it would help to employ the patient's own words and/or rely on open-ended questions to encourage patient collaboration. Knight and von Gunten (2004c) further suggested the use of interfaith language rather than referencing any one religious or spiritual tradition. A desire to be inclusive may be suggested by a reference to "faith community" rather than "church," "religious leader" rather than "priest," and "higher power" rather than "God." As described by Milligan (2011), "Spiritual care begins with encouraging human contact in a compassionate relationship, and moves in whatever direction need requires" (p. 53). The Joint Commission only requires Medicare-certified hospices to complete a spiritual assessment, but the type of spiritual assessment depends on the hospice organization and the professional conducting the assessment (Joint Commission, 2008; NHPCO, n.d.a.). For example, Hodge (2003) described a number of spiritual assessments for social workers; however, these methods have not been evaluated with hospice patients so should be used with caution.

According to Okon (2005), there are two different approaches to spiritual assessment: instrument based and interview based. There is overlap in the spiritual domains addressed by these approaches that includes a patient's experience of, for example, general spirituality, spiritual needs, spiritual coping, and spiritual well-being (Draper, 2012). Instrument-based assessment methods are usually associated with administering measurement tools that are designed to quantify different spiritual dimensions for research purposes. Studies that employ such quantitative measures investigate the association between spiritual dimension(s) and clinical outcome(s). For example, the Spiritual Needs Inventory (Hermann, 2006, 2007) is designed to measure spiritual needs and the Brief RCOPE (Pargament et al., 1998, 2011) is designed to measure religious coping. The Brief RCOPE has been used to test the potential relationship between religious coping and quality of life (Hebert et al., 2009). Using these measures is more time and labor intensive (Milligan, 2011). Such measures are expected to go through a rigorous process of construction, testing, and evaluation by experts to ensure their integrity. For clinical purposes, hospice social workers may employ an interview-based spiritual assessment. This type of spiritual assessment has been described as a spiritual history. For some hospice providers, a spiritual history is a routine part of patient assessment. This approach involves a series of questions for the purposes of capturing a narrative, biographical, or qualitative account of a patient's spiritual life (Draper, 2012). This approach may not result in a lengthy interview or a referral for spiritual care, but it does provide critical information to inform hospice care. A spiritual history may be conducted by using an open-ended format or a structured format.

An Open-Ended Format

A spiritual history with an open format involves questions used to explore a patient's religious and/or spiritual background. As suggested by Okon (2005) and Milligan (2011), hospice social workers may initiate dialogue about spiritual issues by asking "gateway" questions such as:

"Is faith important in your life?"
"What role does spirituality or religion play in your life?"
"Does life feel like a gift or like a burden as you go through this illness?"
"What brings meaning and purpose to your life?"
"In the course of your life, with all its ups and downs, have you found ways of making sense of the things that have happened to you?"
"Are you at peace?"

It is important to employ therapeutic skills such as verbal and nonverbal following and reflection of content and affect. These skills may be used to acknowledge and normalize patient concerns as well as to communicate empathy.

Hodge (2001, 2003, 2005a, 2005b) described how social workers might visually depict spiritual resources in a patient's environment (spiritual ecomap), intergenerational spiritual and religious trends (spiritual genogram), and key moments in a patient's spiritual journey (spiritual life map). For example, as seen in figure 7.1, a spiritual ecomap can be used to depict the strength of a patient's current connection with key aspects associated with a patient's experience of spirituality. These may include religious rituals, God/transcendent, religious community, spiritual leadership, parents' spiritual tradition, and transpersonal beings (e.g., angels or deceased loved ones). Based on Callahan (2015), this ecomap depicts Jo's relationship with social systems that were identified as part of her spiritual history.

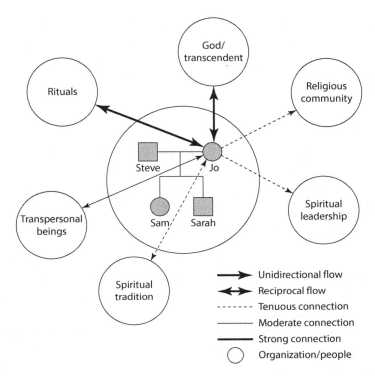

FIGURE 7.1 Example of a spiritual ecomap.

Source: Callahan (2015).

Jo has a tenuous but reciprocal relationship with her spiritual tradition, based on her Catholic upbringing, as it continues to inform her spiritual worldview. Jo also has a tenuous relationship with her church and priest. Even though Jo has sought her church's support, she has had limited contact with church members, since she has been unable to attend church regularly. Jo has a strong, reciprocal relationship with God and relies heavily on religious rituals for spiritual coping. She has a moderate, reciprocal relationship with transpersonal beings identified as her guardian angel, Catholic saints, and the Virgin Mary with whom she connects with through prayer. As suggested by Taylor and Mamier (2004), some patients might not be comfortable with drawing, but this method may provide an alternative approach to communicating spiritual experiences that are too difficult to convey in words (Sessanna et al., 2011).

This also encourages patient collaboration, for the therapeutic narrative should be a "joint construction" process rather than a data-collection process, which is more consistent with an instrument-based approach (Okon, 2005).

A Structured Format

There are many ways a spiritual history may be conducted using a structured format. This approach tends to be the most widely used as part of an admissions assessment (Draper, 2012). According to Okon (2005), these types of formats usually consist of a series of questions that address (1) religious/spiritual/existential beliefs, (2) religious affiliation/membership, (3) what gives meaning and strength, and (4) the impact of beliefs on health-care preferences. Some of these formats employ a mnemonic aide for application. Table 7.2 provides examples of the questions associated with such tools. For example, FICA, which stands for Faith, Importance/Influence, Community, and Address/Action, is a structured format used to conduct a spiritual history (Puchalski & Romer, 2000). Faith could entail asking whether the patient is religious or spiritual. Importance of beliefs in coping with terminal illness would be important to assess. Community affiliation could identify whether a spiritual, religious, or other group is providing patient support. Actions necessary to address a patient's spiritual concerns would identify specific information about how spiritual beliefs may inform hospice care. Draper (2012) suggests a spiritual history should begin with a structured format, because this approach is easy to apply, does not require extensive training, and does not require detailed understanding of different religious or spiritual traditions. The author cautions that since this approach generally does not define spirituality, there is an increased risk for relying on personal assumptions to interpret patient values and preferences. FICA, like similar approaches, was developed based on the general health-care population in the United States. Application with hospice patients of different cultural backgrounds would require additional sensitivity to ensure accurate assessment of patient spiritual needs (Milligan, 2011). Therefore, hospice social workers would need to assess whether the format used is flexible, applicable, nonintrusive, and inclusive (Draper, 2012).

TABLE 7.2   Examples of Structured Formats for Taking a Spiritual History

TOOL	DOMAINS	EXAMPLES OF CONTENT
FICA (Puchalski & Romer, 2000)	**F:** Faith and belief **I:** Importance/influence **C:** Community **A:** Address/action.	**F:** Are there spiritual beliefs that help you cope with stress or difficult times? What gives your life meaning? **I:** Is spirituality important in your life? Are there any particular decisions regarding your health that might be affected by these beliefs? **C:** Are you part of a spiritual or religious community? **A:** Think about what you as the health-care provider need to do with the information the patient shared—e.g., refer to a chaplain, meditation or yoga classes, or another spiritual resource. It helps to be familiar with available resources.
CSI-MEMO (Koenig, 2007)	**C:** Comfort **S:** Stress **I:** Influence **MEM:** Member **O:** Other	**C & S:** Do your religious/spiritual beliefs provide Comfort or are they a source of **Stress**? **I:** Do you have spiritual beliefs that might Influence your medical decisions? **MEM:** Are you a MEMber of a religious or spiritual community and is it supportive of you? **O:** Do you have any Other spiritual needs that you would like someone to address?
HOPE (Anandarajah & Hight, 2001)	**H:** Sources of Hope—meaning, comfort, strength, peace, love and connection **O:** Organized religion **P:** Personal spirituality and practices **E:** Effects on medical care and end-of-life issues	**H:** What is there in your life that gives you internal support? For some people, their religious or spiritual beliefs act as a source of comfort and strength in dealing with life's ups and downs: Is this true for you? If the answer is "Yes," go on to **O** and **P** questions. If the answer is "No," consider asking: Was it ever? If the answer is "Yes," ask: What changed? **O:** Are you part of a religious or spiritual community? Does it help you? How? **P:** Do you have personal spiritual beliefs that are independent of organized religion? What are they? What aspects of your spirituality or spiritual practices do you find most helpful to you personally (e.g., prayer, meditation, reading scripture, attending religious services, listening to music, hiking, communing with nature)?

(continued)

TABLE 7.2   Examples of Structured Formats for Taking a Spiritual History (*Continued*)

TOOL	DOMAINS	EXAMPLES OF CONTENT
		E: Has being sick affected your ability to do the things that usually help you spiritually? (Or affected your relationship with God?) As a hospice social worker, is there anything that I can do to help you access the resources that usually help you? How do your beliefs affect the kind of medical care you would like over the next few days/weeks/months?
SPIRIT (Maugans, 1996)	**S:** Spiritual belief system **P:** Personal spirituality **I:** Integration with a spiritual community **R:** Ritualized practices and Restrictions **I:** Implications for medical care **T:** Terminal events planning	**S:** Name or describe your spiritual belief system. **P:** What does your spirituality/religion mean to you? What is the importance of your spirituality/religion in daily life? **I:** Do you belong to any spiritual or religious group or community? Is it a source of support? In what ways? **R:** Are there specific practices that you carry out as part of your religion/spirituality (e.g., prayer or meditation)? Are there certain lifestyle activities or practices that your religion/spirituality encourages or forbids? Do you comply? **I:** What aspects of your religion/spirituality would you like me to keep in mind as I care for you? **T:** As we plan for your care near the end of life, how does your faith impact your decisions?

When to Consider a Spiritual-Care Referral

Once a spiritual history is complete, it may be determined that a patient's spiritual beliefs and practices are significant resources for coping (Doka, 2011). For example, prayer and being prayed for might be a way a patient feels a meaningful connection to something within and outside of the self. Reliance on rituals and traditions can help sanctify a patient's daily life, maintain a stable routine, and facilitate closure. Patients may read religious scripture or meditate on positive affirmations to gain inspiration. Playing music may cultivate peace. Patients may need family and friends to encourage them by visiting, calling, and sending them cards. A review of current spiritual resources may lead to the identification of new ones or the need to cultivate more, all of which should be documented in a patient's medical record. Interdisciplinary team members can lend insight into patient needs and assist in the referral process (Puchalski et al., 2006). As previously discussed, all hospice social workers can provide implicit spiritual care, but other professionals may be needed to provide explicit spiritual care. A patient's spiritual needs that exceed the hospice social worker's level of expertise necessitate consultation with the spiritual-care provider on the interdisciplinary team team (Okon, 2005), such as hospice chaplains or designated religious/spiritual community leaders. Hospice chaplains can provide both religious and spiritual care, but training varies in the range of interventions chaplains may use to address psychosocial issues (Callahan, 2013; Doka, 2011). As described by Knight and von Gunten (2004c), chaplains may be called at any point while a patient is in hospice care to provide spiritual support. Just like other interdisciplinary team members, chaplains intervene to help patients live life as fully as possible. Chaplains also have the responsibility of providing spiritual support to patients' family members and hospice staff.

Knight and von Gunten (2004c) provided additional resources that included strategies for a successful referral to a hospice chaplain (see box 7.4). Social workers can help patients better understand the role of chaplains. This could reduce the potential for patients to resist referrals. The authors reviewed potential myths a patient might have about chaplains. The myths described by Knight and von Gunten centered on confusion about the role of religion. The authors suggested that patients might believe that chaplains *only* provide religious care. Hospice social workers can confirm that hospice chaplains are often clergy with theological training that enables them to perform religious rites depending on the chaplain's religious affiliation. Chaplains understand how a patient's religious beliefs may influence patient needs for spiritual care. They may provide patients with spiritual resources such as inspirational reading materials. Chaplains also have the training to address a range of spiritual and existential issues. This means chaplains may help patients, for example, explore their core values, ethical concerns, and what gives life meaning to help patients address grief and seek closure (APC, 2015a, 2015b). Knight and von Gunten also suggested that patients might assume a chaplain is a Christian and only serves Christians or

BOX 7.4   STRATEGIES FOR SUCCESSFUL REFERRAL

Referral Strategy #1

Use your own rapport or trust with the patient and family:

"I know this chaplain well and have referred him/her to other patients in my care."

Referral Strategy #2

Offer to set up a meeting or joint visit with the chaplain:

"May I invite him/her to our next appointment?"

"Is it okay if I bring him/her with me this afternoon on rounds?"

Referral Strategy #3

Explain your reasons for suggesting the chaplain and/or indicate your level of concern for the patient's/family's well-being.

"Given how important your religious faith is to you, I think it would be helpful if we asked our chaplain to meet with you before you decide ____."

"I am really concerned about how much suffering you are in and want to be sure you see the person on our staff best equipped to help you. In my opinion that person is ____, our chaplain. He/she can help you much better than I with these important questions you are asking."

Referral Strategy #4

Introduce the chaplain using a description of his or her role rather than the title, if you suspect resistance based upon common misperceptions.

Referral Strategy #5

Consult directly with the chaplain about the needs identified and request her/she stop by the room of the patient or call the patient directly at home. Address confidentiality issues with the patient and family ahead of time so they are prepared to have someone else contacting them who is aware of their condition and needs.

"I will be making other members of our palliative-care team aware of your admission into our program and aware you are considering palliative rather than curative treatment, so they can offer you their assistance directly."

"Our team members include our chaplain and other specialists who will be stopping by to introduce themselves and their services."

From: Knight and von Gunten (2004a).

will try to convert them to a different religion. Hospice social workers can assure patients that hospice chaplains have a professional code of ethics that guides their practice. This includes a respect for all forms of diversity, including religious diversity (APC, 2000, 2004a). Therefore, chaplains recognize that it would be unethical to pressure patients to convert. Chaplains come from different religious backgrounds, some of which are non-Christian. Patients always have the option to request a chaplain with a similar worldview or to work with a religious/spiritual community leader for the spiritual support they prefer.

CONCLUSION

Spiritual sensitivity provides hospice social workers a way to ensure patients gain spiritual support. Spiritual sensitivity requires social workers to balance learner and facilitator roles to enhance the spiritual quality of hospice care (Briggs & Rayle, 2005; Canda & Furman, 1999, 2010). Spiritually sensitive hospice social work is delivered in the same spirit as spiritual care, and encourages personal and professional growth; respect for diverse beliefs, practices, and frameworks for life meaning or worldview; and creative problem solving with the aid of spiritual resources (Briggs & Rayle, 2005; Canda & Furman, 1999, 2010; Krieglstein, 2006). Based on Callahan's (2013, 2015) relational model of spiritually sensitive hospice social work, a therapeutic style of engagement that can enhance a patient's life quality and can, thus, be experienced as meaningful. This experience of enhanced life meaning defines relational spirituality. Spiritual sensitivity can be a form of spiritual care when the provision of hospice social work helps patients meet their spiritual needs. Spiritual care may be indirect, requiring the application of generalist skills, or direct, requiring the application of advanced generalist and/or clinical skills (Callahan, 2015). The type of intervention depends on a patient's spiritual needs and the hospice social worker's expertise, which may require a referral when patient needs extend beyond professional expertise. Hospice social workers may not be responsible for spiritual care but are always responsible for spiritually sensitive care.

The cultivation of relational spirituality through spiritually sensitive hospice social work is congruent with the goals of hospice care to soothe and relieve and spiritual-care goals to inform meaning and purpose. Ongoing spiritual assessment is critical in determining how to engage in spiritually sensitive hospice social work. This clarifies what a patient views as spiritually supportive. To facilitate the delivery of explicit spiritual care, a hospice social worker will need to conduct a spiritual history using an open-ended or structured format. A spiritual history can be used to identify a patient's unmet spiritual needs, experience of spiritual suffering, and access to spiritual resources, and most importantly, whether and how a patient wants to be spiritually supported. The conduct of a spiritual history may be experienced as a form of spiritual care that builds spiritual resilience by empowering patients to collaborate in the process of planning spiritual care. Even though the outcome of a spiritual history may require a referral to a hospice chaplain for spiritual care beyond the scope of hospice social work, the conduct of a spiritual history along with other explicit forms of spiritual care requires an advanced skill set. For a successful referral, hospice social workers might need to address myths patients have about chaplains. The next chapter will focus on how hospice social workers can evaluate the delivery of spiritually sensitive hospice social work based on their level of spiritual competence.

8

Spiritual Competence

SPIRITUALLY SENSITIVE HOSPICE SOCIAL WORK is relational in that it engages patients in a way that respects a patient's individual personhood, dignity, and worth. This type of therapeutic relationship may be a form of spiritual care when it sustains and/or builds spiritual resilience. Although spiritual care can be consoling for patients, it has the potential to be challenging for hospice social workers to negotiate barriers to quality spiritual care. Hospice social workers face the challenge of not only identifying patient spiritual needs but of responding to them in a manner that is congruent with a patient's worldview relative to the hospice social worker's level of professional expertise. This reflects the importance of spiritual competence as supported by research across disciplines and punctuated by the voices of social workers. The building of spiritual competence helps to ensure the delivery of quality spiritual care. Spiritual competence thus provides a means for evaluating the effectiveness of spiritually sensitive hospice social work. The following chapter will describe how spiritual competence enables hospice social workers to be champions of *quality* spiritual care.

CHALLENGES IN PROVIDING SPIRITUAL CARE

Patients have described diverse spiritual needs, and relationships have emerged as a vital resource for the provision of spiritual care. Edwards et al. (2010) found that "spiritual care was not a task or intervention, but was expressed in the way care, including physical care, was given in relationships" (p. 763). The therapeutic power of relationships was affirmed by Langegard and Ahlberg (2009). The authors conducted in-depth interviews with 10 hospice patients with cancer to explore what they had found to be consoling. The experience of connection was one of the ways patients gained a sense of well-being. The types of connection were divided into three subcategories: belonging, communion, and faith in a higher power. Feeling a sense of belonging with family, friends, and caregivers was said to be of greatest importance. Communion with patients who shared a similar diagnosis or were being cared for in the same facility was also said to be comforting. Although communion with family was particularly important, it led to "unbearable" stress when patients struggled to handle stress alone in an effort to protect family members (p. E102). All patients reported the importance of one's relationship with a higher power. Therefore, relationships can provide consolation for hospice patients, but engagement can also lead to professional challenges and personal risk. Langegard and Ahlberg described the experiences of nurses:

> Consoling can be difficult. Words may feel strained and disgenuine [*sic*]. The content may not be what the patient wants to hear, particularly when no possibility of a positive alteration can be recognized. Offering verbal consolation in this situation may not be possible, at least not in the sense of promising the patient future health improvement. The basis for many verbal consolations is that the patient will get better, but, when dealing with a patient with an incurable disease, nurses cannot follow that path. The only recourse is to be a witness . . . a nurse offering consolation should spend time with the suffering patient and communicate that he or she is not alone. A nurse giving consolation must be ready to see and listen to a suffering patient and should, under no circumstances, have any preconceptions, either positive or negative. Feeling safe is a prerequisite in this relationship, for the nurse and the patient. Even in uncertain situations, the nurse should be at the side of the suffering patient. To be receptive and present takes trust. If trust is created, the patient can gather the courage to face the cause of the suffering. The nurse is present at the patient's side and shows that vulnerability, grief, and exposing pain are accepted. Both parties accept that the illness is undeniable, that it exists, and that nothing else can be done . . . A nurse must be open to the patient's suffering in this model; that openness takes courage from both parties.

> (p. E101)

Edwards et al. (2010) examined what patients and palliative-care providers thought were facilitators and barriers to spiritual care. There was an emphasis on having a "friendly spiritual environment" that was conducive for spiritual sharing (p. 763). For patients, this environment was identified as being at home with the support of significant others. Adequate time for palliative-care providers to listen and get to know patients was stressed. Palliative-care providers also noted the importance of having time to connect with interdisciplinary team members to address their own concerns about work. This allowed palliative-care providers to reflect, share, grieve, and find resolution, which included a need to be aware of and cultivate one's own spirituality. Results also revealed barriers to spiritual care. Institutional barriers included high patient numbers, fast turnover, low staffing, large workloads, lack of privacy, and limited funds. It was suggested that an emphasis on task completion resulted in a "loss of the human touch" (p. 763). Spiritual care was described as emotionally challenging and led to compassion fatigue, which was exacerbated by feeling unprepared and having a lack of confidence. Some palliative-care providers noted there was limited access to spiritual-care training. They suggested that addressing diverse spiritual or religious beliefs risked creating an atmosphere of mistrust. However, Edwards et al. said, "Sometimes spirituality was best expressed when there was not a common religion, as it involved sharing common humanity" (p. 763).

Ethical Risks

As suggested by Edwards et al. (2010) and others (Callahan, 2008, 2009a; Coyle, 2001; Grant, 2007; Puchalski, 2013; Puchalski et al., 2006, 2009; Sessanna et al., 2011), hospice social workers face a number of barriers in facilitating quality spiritual care. Barriers to quality spiritual care increase the risk for hospice social workers to engage in boundary crossings and ethical violation. Puchalski et al. (2006) focused on the experience of physicians and nurses, but hospice social workers likely face similar challenges. The authors found that physicians felt they had inadequate time to discuss spiritual issues with patients. They also expressed a desire to avoid discussing spiritual issues, in part because of discomfort with the potential for self-disclosure. Nurses said they lacked time, theoretical knowledge, and training to provide spiritual care. Puchalski et al. suggested that training in the past had encouraged nurses to avoid religious discussions. This might have reduced their sense of responsibility or sanction to provide any form of spiritual care. Having limited time could have been interpreted as a lack of institutional support. Nurses were also at risk for their own spiritual suffering, indicated by a loss of meaning at work, burnout, and desire to withdraw from patients and their families. If the experience of hospice social workers is similar to physicians and nurses, they will need to be prepared to negotiate some significant challenges. Hospice social workers may need to promote institutional conditions that are more supportive of spiritual care. They will also need to build spiritual competence so they themselves are not barriers to quality spiritual care. Overt barriers include proselytizing and other means of influencing patient religious beliefs and practices. Covert barriers may stem from a hospice social worker's unwillingness or inability to provide spiritual care. Hospice social workers can certainly prevent these types of barriers to quality spiritual care.

Coyle (2001) identified overt and covert barriers to quality spiritual care associated with spiritual diversity based on the experience of psychotherapists. Coyle's work suggests that patients might perceive pressure to comply with a hospice social worker's religious/spiritual views, particularly when a hospice social worker's perspective shapes what they consider to be a patient's spiritual needs and/or spiritual resources. There might be efforts by a hospice social worker to influence patient beliefs when they appear to lead to the experience of spiritual suffering, as in the case of negative religious coping described in chapter 4. These circumstances would necessitate consultation with and/or referral to a formal spiritual-care provider. However, in any case, a hospice social worker must offset the risk for patients to feel coerced or rejected based on their religious/spiritual beliefs. Perceived pressure may undermine a patient's core beliefs and values, the loss of which could increase a patient's risk for spiritual suffering. Some patients who feel rejected by a hospice social worker might assume they are likely to be rejected by a divine higher power. Likewise, Sessanna et al. (2011) suggested that a significant barrier to quality spiritual care could involve a failure to respect spiritual diversity. Spiritual assessment and dominant approaches to spiritual care have been shaped by spiritual needs most congruent with Judeo-Christian beliefs. For example, efforts to define spirituality in research have referenced religious affiliation and practices to gauge religious commitment. These approaches may not accurately reflect the experience of patients influenced by Eastern religions or of patients who are spiritual but not religious. Neglecting religion in favor of spirituality, however, risks distorting the experience of people who consider themselves to be both spiritual and religious. Therefore, cultural bias is can influence how hospice social workers approach spiritual assessment, creating a barrier to quality spiritual care (Coyle, 2001; Hodge & Bushfield, 2006).

Need for Spiritual Competence

Ideally, hospice social workers would be facilitators of quality spiritual care. Self-care and professional boundaries that include an awareness of spiritual beliefs, respect for patient diversity, opportunity to debrief with colleagues, and interdisciplinary team collaboration can help facilitate quality spiritual care (Canning et al., 2007; Edwards et al., 2010; Glasper, 2011; Hodge, 2007; NHPCO, 2007). Hodge (2007) indicated that social workers have an ethical responsibility to facilitate spiritual care that is consistent with a patient's worldview. This involves exploring one's own worldview. Glasper (2011) described three ways hospice social workers might express spiritual sensitivity. The first step would be to determine a patient's spiritual needs when providing hospice care. The second step would be to ensure a patient's environment is supportive of spiritual exploration. This might require access to a quite, private space as well as access to a chapel or multifaith room that allows for patient reflection. A spiritually sensitive environment would be one that further values "creativity, flexibility, person-to-person respect, input from all stakeholders in decisions, human development needs, and well-being of the natural environment" (Canda & Furman, 1999, p. 254). The third step would be to develop the spiritual competencies needed to provide spiritual care, assuming the hospice social worker can meet his or her own spiritual needs. For example, a hospice social worker would need self-awareness and clinical judgment to know how to respond when a patient asked for prayer. Glasper said that training was particularly important to be ready for patients uncomfortable with religion and in need of alternative spiritual supports.

Spiritual competence is also necessary for hospice social workers to respond when religion is part of a patient's worldview. Usually, a hospice social worker would refer a patient to a chaplain or other religious/spiritual leader to address religious issues, particularly when a patient's needs extend beyond social work expertise. However, Sulmasy (2009) described how a health-care professional (referenced here as a physician but could also include a hospice social worker) might respond to religious and/or spiritual issues. These four scenarios would likely emerge in the process of delivering hospice social work:

1. When the health-care professional is religious and the patient is also religious, then both should be able to talk about religion in relationship to healing. Some studies have predicted that such concordance in religiosity (but not necessarily in religion) will be the most common situation. The theoretical problems in such cases are only over differences in denomination and in strength of belief.

2. When neither the health-care professional nor the patient is religious, then things might appear to be at their simplest. If neither party is interested in things spiritual, the issue will simply be irrelevant to both parties. However, if the parties do not consider the question irrelevant despite their lack of belief; if they consider themselves spiritual despite their lack of theism, things may be at their most complex. Without any sense of common language or organizing principle for their beliefs, or even rudimentary understanding of the beliefs of the other as an identifiable and organized religion with an accompanying spirituality, it will be extraordinarily difficult to engage in spiritual conversation. They will have to struggle to find a way to speak to each other about their important spiritual concerns. [But with training, the hospice social worker does not need to struggle. Once the hospice social worker knows the patient's worldview, they can draw from that worldview and use the language of the patient (D. Reese, personal communication, February 4, 2016).]

3. When the patient is religious and the health-care professional is not, the physician should take the initiative to make inquiries about the patient's religious beliefs and to be supportive and perhaps even to be encouraging of that patient's beliefs. Even an atheist clinician, who rejects the very possibility of transcendent or spiritual meaning, can know something about various religions and their belief systems and engage patients in fruitful discussions about these beliefs.

4. When the health-care professional is religious and the patient is not, a situation that statistics would predict is the least common of the four scenarios, the situation is most risky with respect to proselytizing . . .

Such clinicians should open up the question of spiritual needs with such patients but then follow the patient's lead in further conversation and inquiry, always respecting the patient's freedom to believe or not to believe.

(p. 8)

The provision of spiritual care that emerges out of these scenarios poses risks for ethical violation and therefore requires a high level of spiritual competence. Usually a chaplain or other formal spiritual-care provider would be required to process religious issues. However, when the interface between religion and spirituality is relevant for patients in the midst of delivering spiritually sensitive hospice social work, advanced generalist/clinical social work intervention could help facilitate spiritual conversations. Intervention should also involve collaboration with interdisciplinary team members, including one's supervisor, to ensure quality spiritual care.

In general, Coyle (2001) suggested that spiritual care should be focused on supporting patient well-being with developmentally appropriate interventions. Emphasis should be on how spirituality supports and is supported by different aspects of a patient's life. Hospice social workers could address universal spiritual themes and should be inclusive rather than focus on the interpretation of religious scripture or theological study. Again, for advanced generalist/clinical social workers this may entail some exploration of religious issues when this informs patient life meaning, but the focus should not be on providing spiritual direction, religious advice, or pastoral counseling. This type of spiritual work would be more appropriate for hospice chaplains, spiritual leaders, or related representatives (Hodge, 2011). Puchalski (2013) suggests the following guidelines that would further help hospice social workers:

1. Operate from a broad definition of spirituality.
2. Use professional boundaries that maintain a patient's trust.
3. Conduct a patient-centered spiritual assessment.
4. Avoid attempting to answer unanswerable questions such as "Why me?"
5. Avoid religious proselytizing, inappropriate persuasion, or giving spiritual advice.
6. Rely on patients to direct prayer.
7. Avoid spiritual care outside competence.
8. Consult with hospice chaplains and other spiritual leaders for guidance.

It is essential for hospice social workers to seek additional training to build spiritual competence. This can inspire confidence in one's ability to deliver quality spiritual care (Coyle, 2001). Likewise, the ability to determine one's level of spiritual competence provides a way to evaluate spiritually sensitive hospice social work. Conversely, without spiritual competence, there is a risk of neglecting a patient's spiritual needs and even violating a patient's spiritual boundaries.

DEFINING SPIRITUAL COMPETENCE

Terminal illness may be considered a life event that can lead to profound changes, some of which are unique or experienced differently relative to each person. Spirituality along with race, gender, age, ethnicity, ability, sexual orientation, and gender identity are among the many factors that define personhood, including a person's worldview. Hospice social workers are expected to be aware of how diverse biopsychosocial-spiritual factors contribute to a patient's well-being. As described in chapter 1, the *Code of Ethics of the National Association of Social Workers* (NASW, 2008), *NASW Standards for Social Work Practice in Palliative and End of Life* (2004), and *Indicators for the Achievement of the NASW Standards for Cultural Competence in Social Work Practice* (2001, 2015) all stress the importance of cultural competence. The Council on Social Work Education (CSWE) *Educational Policy and Accreditation Standards* (2008; 2015a) further require social work programs to build spiritual competence. Spiritual competence is considered a more specific form of cultural competence (Hodge et al., 2006; Hodge & Bushfield, 2006). Competence is associated with the ability to employ skills that reflect professional values, attitudes, and knowledge (Wintz, 2004). Professional competencies provide a way hospice social workers can evaluate sensitivity to spiritual diversity and, likewise, the delivery of spiritually sensitive hospice social work.

As part of the CSWE (2015b, 2015c), the Religion and Spirituality Work Group was created in 2011 to help social workers learn more about diverse expressions of spirituality. This Work Group operates an online clearinghouse of information that can help social workers learn more about spiritually competent practice. As described by the group's mission:

Given the pervasiveness of religion and spirituality throughout people's lives and cultures, social workers need to understand religion and spirituality to develop a holistic view of the person in environment and to support the professional mission of promoting satisfaction of basic needs, well-being, and justice for all individuals and communities around the world.

(p. 2)

Hospice social workers are responsible for operating in a manner that is sensitive to a patient's spiritual needs for spirituality can have implications for one's life quality. Models of spiritual competence provide a way to evaluate the delivery of spiritually sensitive hospice social work. This approach assumes that it is not possible to be spiritually competent without being spiritually sensitive (D. Hodge, personal communication, November 1, 2013). Being spiritually insensitive could, thus, involve behaviors previously mentioned that inhibit patient access to quality spiritual care. Spiritual competence has been described as ranging on a continuum, with a lack of spiritual competence suggesting spiritual insensitivity and, in some cases, spiritually destructive practices on the opposite end of the continuum (Hodge et al., 2006). Hence, a lack of spiritual competence can translate into behaviors that harm patients.

The importance of spiritual competence is reflected in models developed across disciplines and practice settings. As summarized in table 8.1, the work of Hodge (2011) and associates (Hodge & Bushfield, 2006; Hodge et al., 2006) and the SSSW (n.d.) describes spiritually competent practices that are expected as part of the delivery of generalist interventions. Additional work by the Association for Spiritual, Ethical, and Religious Values in Counseling (ASERVIC, 2009) identified spiritual competencies that are endorsed by the American Counseling Association. These competencies are similar to those of the SSSW but are more specific to psychotherapeutic interventions in line with advanced generalist/clinical interventions. Taken together, these guidelines for spiritual competence can be used to evaluate the quality of spiritual care in hospice- and palliative-care settings. To summarize, the following discussion will rely on Hodge (2011) and associates (Hodge & Bushfield, 2006; Hodge et al., 2006) but will return to the interdisciplinary model of spiritual care by Puchalski et al. (2009) to review the importance of collaboration.

TABLE 8.1 Spiritual Competency Models across Disciplines and Practice Settings

Hodge (2011) and Hodge and Bushfield (2006): Spiritual competence as defined by self-awareness, empathic understanding of clients, and use of evidence-based interventions	SSSW (n.d.): Spiritual competence as defined by values and attitudes, knowledge, and skills	Cooper, Aheme, and Pereira (2009): Spiritual competence as defined by characteristics, knowledge, and skills	ASERVIC (2009): Spiritual competence as defined by self-awareness, knowledge of client worldview and development, and spiritually sensitive interventions	Puchalski et al. (2009): Spiritual competence as defined by values and collaboration with patients, families, and health- and spiritual-care professionals
Awareness of personal worldview and related assumptions	**Values and attitudes** • Use a nonjudgmental approach around spiritual issues • Value and respect diversity • Affirm and support spiritualities different from self • Support client self-determination • Represent clinical, social, or ethical perspectives that may support or conflict with a client's worldview respectfully and with integrity	**Characteristics** • Sensitivity • Sensibility to a range of circumstances, family contexts, and traditions and how those interact in complex end-of-life care situations • Compassionate • Covenant-based presence[1] • Nonjudgmental • Reflective practitioner • Ability to contain/tolerate ambiguity • Tolerance for sadness • Courage for moving into the suffering of others • Humility (no easy answers/quick solutions) • mutual search for meaning • Trust that meaning within chaos/suffering exists[2]	**Self-awareness** • Actively explore one's own attitudes, beliefs, and values about spirituality and/or religion • Evaluate the influence of one's own spiritual and/or religious beliefs and values on the client and the counseling process • Identify the limits of one's understanding of the client's spiritual and/or religious perspective and be acquainted with religious and spiritual resources and leaders who can be avenues for consultation and to whom the counselor can refer	**Values** • Autonomy, compassion, competence, courage, dignity, equality, generosity, humility, integrity, justice, respect, reverence, trust, and worth of patients

	Knowledge	Knowledge	Knowledge	Skills	Skills
Empathic understanding of client worldview	• Major faith traditions and the variety of spiritual experiences they support • Social context of spiritual experience, and how culture interacts with spirituality • Alternative expressions of spirituality • Dynamics of change, and how spirituality contributes to the change process • Current issues affecting and affected by spirituality (abortion, LGBTQ issues, death penalty, domestic violence)	• Range of religious traditions and rituals/rites • Flags for a range of "abuse" circumstances/history • Major non-Western cultural considerations/"flags" in your catchment (e.g., taboos, ambiguities) • Bioethical decision frameworks • Grief and bereavement theory and practices • Family dynamics theory • Self-care strategies • Conflict management theory and practices • Service and program development models and practices • Organizational dynamics in large health-care environments • Constructs of "being," "hope," "suffering," and "redemption" • Assessment/protocols appropriate to spiritual care	**Culture and worldview** • Describe the similarities and differences between spirituality and religion, including the basic beliefs of various spiritual systems, major world religions, agnosticism, and atheism • Recognize that the client's beliefs (or absence of beliefs) about spirituality and/or religion are central to his or her worldview and can influence psychosocial functioning **Human and spiritual development** • Can describe and apply various models of spiritual and/or religious development and their relationship to human development	• Take and write a spiritual history • Assess an individual client's relationship to a faith tradition or other body of spiritual practice • Assess spiritual strengths and barriers as they support or impede a desired change	
Evidence-based intervention Interventions must be based on: • Client's preferences • Clinical expertise				• Leadership in ethical decision making • Patient advocacy and "interests" representation • Mediation • "Boundary" management in personal, family, and interprofessional/provider relations • Generic negotiation skills	**Communication** • Respond to client communications about spirituality and/or religion with acceptance and sensitivity • Use spiritual and/or religious concepts that are consistent with the client's spiritual and/or religious perspectives and are acceptable to the client **Intervention** • Recognize spirituality as an integral component to the human experience of ill-ness, healing, and health • Perform spiritual inquiry in a patient-centered, confidential, and respectful manner

(continued)

TABLE 8.1 Spiritual Competency Models across Disciplines and Practice Settings (*Continued*)

• Relevant research • Cultural competency	• Assess what spiritual resources would be appropriate to a client's case plan • Identify and procure spiritually competent resources as needed • Identify points of divergence and convergence in the helping relationship and draw appropriate boundaries around them • Include spiritually informed interventions that are appropriate to the client and the situation • Select and practice self-care activities that support the social worker's work without infringing on the rights or sensibilities of one's clients or co-workers	• Active listening and restating/rephrasing for confirmation of understanding • Empathic listening • Asking open questions to invite open responses for building understanding • Generic counseling skills applied to several different circumstances • Coordination of people/resources within different care settings • Teamwork and team building • Effective teaching-learning strategies and methods • Brokering of diverse interests • Generic crisis intervention skills applied to a variety of contexts • Modeling humanistic and compassionate behavior • Consultative skills	• Recognize spiritual and/or religious themes in client communication and be able to address these with the client when they are therapeutically relevant **Assessment** • During intake and assessment, strive to understand a client's spiritual and/or religious perspective by gathering information from the client and/or other sources **Diagnosis and treatment** • When making a diagnosis, recognize that the client's spiritual and/or religious perspectives can (1) enhance well-being; (2) contribute to client problems; and/or (3) exacerbate symptoms • Set goals with the client that are consistent with the client's spiritual and/or religious perspectives • Able to (1) modify therapeutic techniques to include a client's spiritual and/or religious perspectives, and (2) utilize spiritual and/or religious practices as techniques when appropriate and acceptable to a client's viewpoint • Can therapeutically apply theory and current research supporting the inclusion of a client's spiritual and/or religious perspectives and practices	• Elicit the patient's ongoing spiritual concerns/issues/needs • Be sensitive to the ways in which a patient describes spiritual beliefs, practices, values, meaning, and relationships • Respect patient autonomy to address or not address spirituality • Practice spiritual self-care as a provider of spiritual care • Collaborate with qualified interdisciplinary professionals • Provide competent and compassionate spiritual care • Work in partnership in the study, application, and advancement of scientific knowledge regarding spirituality and health care • Perform only those services for which one is qualified, observe all laws, and uphold the dignity and honor of one's profession

[1] The authors noted that this characteristic may not be clearly understood.
[2] The authors noted that this characteristic may not be universally applicable.

A SOCIAL WORK MODEL OF SPIRITUAL COMPETENCE

According to Hodge and Bushfield (2006), spiritual competence consists of three dimensions that "overlap, inform, and build upon one another" (p. 106). The building of spiritual competence is expected to be a continuous process. This process includes building an awareness of personal worldview and assumptions, empathic understanding of a patient's worldview, and interventions that are sensitive to a patient's worldview (Hodge, 2011; Hodge et al., 2006; Hodge & Bushfield, 2006). This worldview may not be religious. It may not be considered by the patient as spiritual either, but hospice social workers will need to assess what informs a patient's life meaning.

Awareness of Personal Worldview

Every person has particular qualities that are self-defining. Some of these qualities, as mentioned earlier, include race, gender, age, and ethnicity. Personal values and beliefs are among those factors that not only shape a patient's worldview but also a hospice social worker's worldview. Some of these values and beliefs may be embraced intentionally, such as a religious affiliation, while others may not, as they are acquired through socialization. Values and beliefs also define a hospice social worker's worldview, further shaping professional practice. Given the power differential inherent in a therapeutic relationship and likelihood of working with populations at risk for discrimination, it is important for hospice social workers to be self-aware. As described by Hodge (2011), self-awareness can help social workers manage the potential for "spiritual countertransference," which entails imposing one's own spiritual concerns, values, or beliefs onto patients (p. 154). Hospice social workers can benefit from understanding how one's definition of spirituality, including religion, may be different from a patient's definition of spirituality. This can inspire respect for spiritual diversity and influence one's sense of comfort in addressing spirituality with patients (Callahan, 2011d; Callahan, Benner, & Helton, 2016).

Empathic Understanding of a Patient's Worldview

It is likewise important to learn about the spiritual values and beliefs that inform a patient's worldview, particularly when patients are from backgrounds unfamiliar to the hospice social worker. As described by Hodge and Bushfield (2006), it is not necessary to share similar spiritual values and beliefs, but it is necessary to respect diversity and approach such differences as being as legitimate as one's own. This includes operating with an awareness of a patient's spiritual strengths and resources, which may require additional efforts to seek information about a patient's religious or spiritual background. It is important to note that diversity is likely to exist within a single religious or spiritual tradition, as patients may ascribe to beliefs that are not congruent with the norm (Hodge, 2011). As suggested by Hodge (2011), social workers can learn about different traditions by visiting houses of worship, reading related materials, talking with congregants/religious leaders, and consulting with interdisciplinary team members. This may involve patient referral to professional with a higher level of spiritual competence.

Use of Evidence-Based Interventions

Hospice social workers need the ability to engage in generalist and advanced generalist/clinical interventions that are congruent with a patient's worldview. Drawing from spiritual resources identified by a patient and those that are within the patient's ability to utilize can build trust and stimulate motivation for spiritual self-care. There are also times when spiritual care may be contraindicated. According to Hodge (2011), spiritual care may not always be appropriate particularly when spirituality is unrelated to patient issues, patients are not interested in addressing spiritual issues, there is not enough information available to guide intervention, or the hospice social worker lacks the expertise to intervene. Spiritual care should not be facilitated with minors without consent of a parent or legal guardian. Poor application of spiritual care can exacerbate rather than ameliorate suffering. It is essential to balance respect for patient beliefs and practices with change oriented strategies that promote spiritual resilience. Hospice social workers may help patients identify new resources or the need to cultivate more. Hodge (2011) further suggested that evidence-based practice would require an awareness of a hospice patient's preferences, relevant research, clinical expertise, and cultural competence.

PATIENT PREFERENCES

Spiritually sensitive hospice social work is patient centered, and so it is essential to understand a patient's preferences for spiritual care. This can be difficult without a spiritual assessment. Since spirituality is a fluctuating state, and spiritual needs may change throughout the duration of care, ongoing spiritual assessment will be necessary. A formal spiritual history depends on a patient's willingness to participate and presupposes hospice social workers have the expertise to engage in this advanced generalist/clinical intervention. As described in chapter 7, assessment starts with the collection of basic information about the patient. This may include gateway questions that capture a patient's interest in addressing spirituality. According to Koenig (2007), the extent of assessment may consist of a single question such as "Do you have any spiritual needs or concerns related to your health?" (p. 44). If a patient expresses spiritual needs or concerns, then a spiritual history may ensue to clarify spiritual-care preferences and resources. This may entail support from interdisciplinary team members with more experience or additional information to complete the assessment. A spiritual history should be prefaced with disclosure of purpose to ensure respect for patient preferences and elicit patient consent, treatment collaboration, and likelihood of success (Hodge, 2011). To identify the types of preferences a patient may have for spiritual care, it may help to reference the spiritual needs a patient presents with based on palliative- and hospice-care research.

For example, Edwards et al. (2010) conducted a meta-analysis of qualitative research that included 11 studies based on interviews hospice patients (n = 178) about spirituality. These patients were mainly white with Judeo-Christian religious backgrounds and had been diagnosed with cancer. Results indicated that they wanted professional caregivers to be compassionate, kind, gentle, and comforting. Patients wanted to feel loved, affirmed, valued, and nurtured by professional caregivers as human beings worthy of respect and dignity. They wanted a sense of belonging and to have support for their worldviews. Patients wanted choice in shaping the direction of care, with a preference for maintaining the ordinariness of life at home. In terms of the qualities of the caregiving relationship, patients wanted good rapport that instilled trust and boundaries that were flexible enough for reciprocal sharing. They wanted someone to help them face their illness as a companion and guide and to act as a support for their family members. Patients wanted professional caregivers to create the conditions that helped them feel more comfortable in expressing their spiritual concerns. This entailed active listening, open questions, and communication of empathy. They wanted to be able to meet their own spiritual needs. Some patients used art and music to express feelings that were too difficult to verbalize. Drawing from box 8.1, originally referenced in chapter 7, spiritual-care interventions patients preferred as reported in Edwards et al. were compared with other research, some of which did not focus on patient reports. Interventions in italics were not reported by patients in the Edwards et al. study. Such disparity is a reminder of the importance of asking patients what they want and need, because it may be different from what others say.

CLINICAL EXPERTISE

Before engaging in the delivery of spiritual care, hospice social workers should consider the level of spiritual competence necessary for ethical practice (Hodge, 2011; NASW, 2008). This includes reflecting on how one might respond to ethical challenges, some of which are found in box 8.2. Social work education and experience provide a basic level of spiritual competence for generalist interventions. There is also a growing body of literature, professional conferences, and presentations/workshops to build spiritual competence for advanced generalist/clinical interventions. Knight and von Gunten (2004a) offered questions a hospice social worker might consider before engaging in intervention:

- Do I know how to assess whether this patient's "pain" is physical or spiritual in origin?
- Am I comfortable talking with this family about their religious beliefs and practices?
- Am I likely to impose my own set of values or beliefs upon them in the process of assessing their needs?
- Will I be comfortable in the face of strong emotions that may arise in the process of a more in-depth assessment of spiritual suffering?
- Will I have the time and skills to provide comfort if my questions evoke great sadness or distress?
- Who could best meet the needs of this patient and family at this time?

(n.p.)

If a hospice social worker does not have the appropriate level of expertise, consultation with interdisciplinary team members with more experience would be necessary. Hospice programs are likely to have chaplains, but there also may be other spiritual leaders or related representatives in the community who may be identified by a patient. Additional steps may be required to facilitate a referral, particularly if a patient has some reservations about drawing from alternative resources. This is when hospice social workers may need to educate patients about the role of chaplains as being professionals with expertise to help patients address questions about core values and ethical issues (Knight & von Gunten, 2004a).

BOX 8.1   EXAMPLES OF SPIRITUAL-CARE INTERVENTIONS

Generalist Interventions

Modes of delivery: therapeutic relationship, psycho-education, and supportive counseling (individual, family, and group)

1. Being compassionate
2. Being empathic/*relating/understanding*
3. Evidencing trustworthiness
4. Being affirming/valuing/respecting patient dignity/supporting/*accepting/ positive regard/humanizing/validating*
5. Being kind/gentle/comforting/loving/nurturing/*caring/warm/attending*
6. Being a companion/patient-centered/*providing personalized support/recognizing uniqueness/collaborative*
7. Facilitating relationships
8. Focusing on the ordinariness of life
9. Maintaining good rapport/asking open questions/*communicating skillfully*
10. *Expressing a genuine desire to understand/enjoying time together*
11. *Being present or available/connecting/offering a therapeutic touch/promising nonabandonment/being a witness to the patient's experience/accompanying the patient on this journey*
12. Active listening/*using silence effectively*
13. *Having self-awareness and spiritual knowing*
14. Making a referral

Advanced Generalist/Clinical Interventions

Modes of delivery: therapeutic relationship, psycho-education, psychotherapy (individual, family, and group), and alternative:*

1. *Completing a spiritual assessment*
2. Facilitating spiritual expression/*spiritual conversations*
3. Setting flexible boundaries/offering reciprocal sharing

BOX 8.1 EXAMPLES OF SPIRITUAL-CARE INTERVENTIONS (CONTINUED)

4. Providing guidance/*problem solving*
5. Enabling spiritual self-care/*identifying inner resources/supporting personal belief systems*
6. *Identifying potential spiritual/religious resources*
7. *Offering bereavement counseling/end-of-life planning*
8. *Aiding in life review/listening to reminiscences/enabling meaning making/ identifying ways to make memories*
9. *Inspiring hope*
10. *Reframing*
11. *Using humor*

*Alternative modes of delivery include art therapy, music therapy, *dream work*, acupuncture, therapeutic touch, biofeedback, relaxation response, guided imagery, and aromatherapy.

Sources: Byock, 1996; Carroll, 2001; Cavendish et al., 2003; Chaturvedi, 2007; Chochinov & Cann, 2005; Cornette, 2005; Edwards et al., 2010; Exline et al., 2013; Ferrell, 2011; Glasper, 2011; Heyse-Moore, 1996; Hills et al., 2005; HPNA, 2013; Kisvetrova, Kluger, & Kabelka, 2013; Mako et al., 2006; Milligan, 2011; Mitchell et al., 2006; Narayanasamy, 2007; NHPCO, 2007; Okon, 2005; Penman et al., 2007; Puchalski, 2008a, 2008b, 2008c, 2013; Puchalski et al., 2006, 2009; Sperry, 2010; Sperry & Miller, 2010; Stern & James, 2006.

BOX 8.2 ANTICIPATING ETHICAL DILEMMAS

Scenario 1

Question: Would you provide spiritual care without adequate time for follow-up if the patient was in the midst of spiritual distress without immediate support?

I was working with a patient who was struggling with her terminal illness. The family was present. I could tell she was having a hard time. Finally I asked her, "Are you scared?" She started crying and we had a pretty good session, but I was unable to follow-up for 3 weeks, given the number of other people I needed to see. The family said, "Where are you?," and they found resource reasons to bring me back there.

Response: A referral to a chaplain would have been appropriate. A chaplain would have had official sanction to devote more time to address the spiritual suffering suggested by the patient's fear of death. A chaplain might have also reduced the need for the patient and family to find "resource reasons" to justify having the hospice social worker follow up.

BOX 8.2 (CONTINUED)

Scenario 2

Question: Would you avoid a referral to a chaplain or formal spiritual-care provider if you think you can address the patient's spiritual needs?

I had a patient who said that he had walked with the Lord, but had become very bitter. He began to cry, and it turned into a spiritual conversation. He began to talk about why he was so angry at his church. It was because he had done so many things there, and in his dying days he felt like they left him when he needed them. He told me because I had the time to listen.

Response: Giving the immediacy of the patient's need to talk, it was appropriate to take the time to listen. In this case, the hospice social worker should also ask whether the patient would like a referral to a chaplain or for someone in the patient's church to be contacted. This could have helped the patient resolve feelings of abandonment by his church (and, perhaps, God).

Scenario 3

Question: Would you offer or make a referral to a chaplain or formal spiritual-care provider if you did not believe the chaplain would respect patient beliefs?

There can be a lot of shame for patients when a chaplain goes in. If he isn't trying to save this person, the chaplain thinks he isn't doing his job. I wish our chaplains were more trained. They may assume the role of chaplain without a lot of seminary training. The more trained they are, the better they are in dealing with all different kinds of beliefs.

Response: It is important to determine whether it is in the best interests of the patient to offer a referral to a chaplain. Although it is an ethical violation for chaplains to proselytize, some chaplains may not be board certified, and seminary training blurs professional roles. There may be a different formal spiritual-care provider with more expertise. The patient and/or family members may also prefer to rely on someone else they trust. This may include the social worker with the capacity to provide ongoing spiritual support.

Scenario 4

Question: Would you pray for/with a patient if you felt certain you or the patient would suffer enduring spiritual consequences?

I pray with them. I hold their hand and say, "Do you want me to pray? Squeeze my hand if you do. If you have accepted Christ, squeeze my hand." If they have not

BOX 8.2 (CONTINUED)

already accepted Christ and want to, I will pray the prayer of salvation. Then I will ask, "If you feel peace in your heart, please squeeze my hand." Many times I have had that happen. They are at peace.

Response: It is never appropriate to proselytize as a hospice social worker. Any prayer with a patient should be one that is directed by the patient. If the patient insists on the hospice social worker leading the prayer, the prayer should be brief and inclusive. The hospice social worker may also rely on the spiritual language used by the patient if they need to be more specific.

Scenario 5

Question: Would you pray for/with a patient without securing reliable and clear patient consent for spiritual care?

I pray silently for patients while providing them hospice care if it seems the patient does not share similar religious beliefs that would allow for direct provision of spiritual care.

Response: Although private prayer cannot be regulated, praying for a patient violates the rights of patients who might be uncomfortable or would likely refuse spiritual care, including prayer. Alternatively, a hospice social worker may focus prayer to support one's own spiritual growth or to cope with challenging work conditions.

Source: Callahan (2011c).

RELEVANT RESEARCH

It is important for hospice social workers to be aware of the best available research on spiritual care with patients nearing the end of life. What is considered the best available research is relative to the type of information needed and research methods employed. There are different frameworks that classify some research as being more scientifically credible than others. In general, scientifically credible research is likely to be found in peer-reviewed journals. Systematic reviews or meta-analyses would be the most reliable way to gain a broad understanding of the literature. In the process, it is important to consider the worldview of the researcher and types of patients included in the studies reviewed. For example, results from in-depth qualitative interviews with a few patients only represent the experience of those patients. As Hodge (2011) warned, "Interventions developed, tested, and validated with one cultural group may not prove effective with another, so too, interventions that are effective with one spiritual population may not be effective with another because of differences in how the populations construct reality" (p. 152). Studies with large sample sizes that employ both qualitative and quantitative measures to analyze patient experiences may have wider application but may lack depth of exploration and fail to truly capture the spiritual dimensions of an experience. Hence, all available research should be considered (Hodge, 2011). It is also important to consider how one's own perspective might influence the interpretation of research. Information may be gleaned through other resources, such as books, professional conferences, and presentations/workshops. Consider the background of the author, publisher, or sponsor when evaluating credibility. Just because a professional body sponsors a presentation does not mean the presenter's information is accurate.

CULTURAL COMPETENCE

Hodge (2011) and Hodge and Bushfield (2006) focus on the concept of spiritual competence, but likewise encourage a broader level of cultural competence since cultural diversity shapes daily experiences, including the provision of hospice social work. Cultural diversity is most often associated with demographic differences due to race, gender, age, religion, ethnicity, ability, and sexual orientation. These individual factors are referenced to help shape one's identity. The intersection of these differences requires additional awareness of how identification with a single and/or multiple identities may shape an individual's worldview. This entails experiences that are distinct from identifying with a particular religious and/or spiritual tradition, such as a lifetime of racial discrimination. As seen in table 8.2, Fukuyama and Sevig (1999) and Baggs, Wolf, Puig, and Fukuyama (2009) suggested that spiritual competence and cultural competence are related but different constructs. Similar to spiritual competence, cultural competence requires social workers to be self-aware and make efforts to understand how minority cultures operate. For example, African Americans are more likely to rely on family support and prayer to sustain hope in a miracle rather than to choose hospice care. They are more likely to tolerate pain,

TABLE 8.2   Conceptual Connections but Distinct Competencies

COMPETENCIES	SPIRITUAL COMPETENCE	CULTURAL COMPETENCE
Personal awareness	What are my spiritual beliefs and how do they affect others?	What is the impact of my social identity group membership?
Knowledge	Do I know about various religions and spiritual philosophies?	Can I recognize the history of oppression?
Skills	Can I recognize group dynamics that include spiritual issues?	Can I recognize group dynamics that include multicultural issues?
Passion	Can I communicate compassion and love?	Can I communicate understanding and empathy?
Action	Can I demonstrate acceptance of a variety of religious and spiritual beliefs?	Can I take proactive measures against oppression?

Adapted from: Baggs et al. (2009) and Fukuyama & Sevig (1999).

given spiritual value associated with suffering, but African Americans are also likely to accept death as God's will and use funeral rites as a celebration of life (Callahan, 2015; Reese et al., 2010). While it is important to identify cultural strengths that moderate systemic oppression, spirituality may or may not be a defining factor for an individual patient regardless of cultural norms. Cultural competence thus ensures hospice care communicates respect for individual diversity within and across cultural groups.

ADDITIONAL STEPS FOR EVALUATION

To engage in spiritually sensitive hospice social, a social worker must operate within his or her level of spiritual competence; otherwise, the hospice social worker and intervention would fail to be spiritually sensitive. Therefore, guidelines for spiritual competence provide a foundation for spiritual care delivery and evaluation. It can be challenging to assess the delivery of spiritual care, and likewise, spiritually sensitive hospice social work, since spirituality can be a fluctuating state. To evaluate success in spiritually sensitive hospice social work, there must be evidence that a patient has been positively changed by the therapeutic relationship, which is associated with the experience of relational spirituality. To more specifically evaluate success in spiritual care, there should be evidence that a patient's spiritual needs, such as the experience of joy in rekindling a meaningful relationship, have been met. Spiritual resilience may be indicated by a patient's discovery of new meaning through spiritual practices. Just like other social work interventions, patient needs help determine goals and objectives for spiritual care. Hospice social workers should rely on patient observation and report to help determine success. The perspectives of loved ones, community members, and interdisciplinary team members may help. The time involved to arrange a full evaluation, however, may not be feasible, and so a hospice social worker should continually assess his or her level of spiritual competence. Narayanasamy (2007) proposes the following questions for preliminary evaluation of spiritual care:

1. Is the patient's belief system stronger?
2. Do the patient's professed beliefs support and direct actions and words?
3. Does the patient gain peace and strength from spiritual resources (such as prayer and minister's visits) to face the rigors of treatment, rehabilitation or peaceful death?
4. Does the patient seem more in control and have a clearer self-concept?
5. Is the patient at ease in being alone and in having life plans changed?
6. Is the patient's behavior appropriate to the occasion?
7. Has reconciliation of any differences taken place between the patient and others?
8. Are mutual respect and love obvious in the patient's relationships with others?
9. Are there any signs of physical improvement?
10. Is there an improved rapport with other patients?

(pp. 8–9)

Quantitative methods for assessing the quality of spiritual care may include rates of completing spiritual assessments, numbers of chaplain referrals, inclusion of spiritual resources in treatment plans, and scores on spiritual measures (Puchalski et al., 2009). For example, the Social Work Assessment Tool (SWAT) by Reese et al. (2006) could be used to evaluate how well a patient is doing spiritually on a scale from 1 to 5, along with 11

other dimensions, after each session. Examples of other issues include sui-
cidal ideation, death anxiety, and social support (see http://www.nhpco
.org/sites/default/files/public/nchpp/SWAT_Information_Booklet
.pdf). This allows the hospice social worker to reflect on how well a
patient is doing spiritually in comparison with other issues addressed as
part of hospice social work. There is also a version of SWAT in which
patients can rate themselves and a primary-caregiver version. Hospice
social workers can compare the results to evaluate progress over time.
Although the SWAT may not be sensitive enough to measure a patient's
experience of enhanced life meaning, it does provide a preliminary
way to document how a patient is doing spiritually in effort to evaluate the quality of spiritual care. Ideally, however, a full evaluation with
both qualitative and quantitative methods would be best to determine
whether spiritually sensitive hospice social work is an effective way to
deliver spiritual care.

INTERPROFESSIONAL COLLABORATION

Puchalski et al. (2009) indicated that the national standard for spiritual
care is a collaborative process that supports patient spirituality throughout the trajectory of illness. As described in chapter 1, in 2001 the NCP
(2015) was founded by national leaders "to create clinical practice guidelines that improve the quality of palliative care in the United States" (p. 1).
These voluntary guidelines are the product of the work of interdisciplinary
experts and professional organizations. The NCP's *Clinical Practice Guidelines for Quality Palliative Care* was published in 2004. These guidelines
have been endorsed by many organizations, including the NASW and
the SWHPN. In 2006, the NCP worked with the NQF, to develop preferred practices based on research that can be used to inform measurable
outcomes for hospice social workers (NQF, 2006; NCP, 2013). The NCP
guidelines were later revised, and a second edition was published in 2009,
with the third and most recent edition released in 2013. These documents
provide information about the spiritual, religious, and existential aspects
of care (see box 1.2 on p. 29). A desire to support the provision of quality
spiritual care also led to a national consensus conference in 2009.

Puchalski et al. (2009) built upon the 2009 NCP guidelines, NQF preferred practices, and consensus conference proceedings to summarize key

aspects of spiritual care. Their report highlights the importance of interprofessional collaboration. It is through interprofessional collaboration that hospice social workers can serve as valuable resources for both patients and team members. The authors recognized that it would not be possible for one professional to meet every biopsychosocial and spiritual need, but interdisciplinary team members could share in this responsibility to patients. As recommended by Puchalski et al.:

> Initial screening and some treatment of spiritual issues may be done by health care professionals such as physicians, counselors, parish nurses, and social workers. More complex spiritual issues [particularly religious issues that may necessitate theological expertise and religious rites] need to be attended to by a board-certified chaplain or equivalently prepared spiritual care provider.
>
> (p. 899)

The benefit of an interdisciplinary team is the ability to apportion roles that fall within one's professional expertise. BCCs are most directly responsible for spiritual care and may serve as spiritual care coordinators. When a hospice chaplain is not available, Puchalski et al. suggested, "Physicians and advance practice nurses can consult with social workers and outpatient chaplains or other equivalently trained spiritual care professionals" (p. 898). Thus, it is assumed that hospice social workers have the spiritual competence and confidence to assist interdisciplinary team members. Depending on available resources, hospice social workers might be the primary providers of spiritual care.

As part of delivering quality spiritual care, interprofessional collaboration requires respect for the expertise of interdisciplinary team members as well as maintenance of professional team dynamics. Communication through team meetings, documentation of spiritual concerns in the patient record, and contribution toward treatment plans are all critical components of interprofessional collaboration. Team dynamics should not sacrifice professional integrity for team harmony, but interdisciplinary team members should support a healing environment. This may entail efforts to facilitate activities and programs to build compassion and respect. Puchalski et al. suggested that "in addition to social workers, chaplains, physicians, and nurses, there are other spiritual professionals who can participate as part of the larger palliative care team" (p. 899). These extended team members are people in the community such as volunteer chaplains, religious leaders, members of faith communities, culturally based healers, pastoral counselors, spiritual directors, and other spiritual-care providers. Ideally, interdisciplinary team members would be able to assess a volunteer's preparation to be a spiritual resource. Therefore, through interdisciplinary collaboration backed by evidence-based practice, spiritual care *can* be delivered as a fundamental component of quality palliative and hospice care.

CONCLUSION

There are special qualities in the relationship between a hospice social worker and patient. There can be a deep sense of intimacy in being involved with patients that requires restraint, compassion, and confidentiality. Patients who are dying may feel very little control over their lives and perceive hospice social workers as having tremendous power. This inherent power differential necessitates particular qualities and skills to ensure patient needs are respected, including spiritual needs. The vulnerability of hospice patients further poses an ethical obligation to be spiritually competent. As asserted by Puchalski et al. (2009), quality hospice and palliative care requires spiritual needs to be addressed throughout the trajectory of illness, beginning at the time of diagnosis. Professional boundaries reduce the risk for ethical violations that can result when hospice social workers are stressed, overworked, or struggling with loss. Skillful spiritual care can create a safe spiritual space for patients nearing the end of life, one that is free from proselytizing or other forms of spiritual coercion. Spiritual care is not intended to provide answers to unanswerable questions but to open a spiritual dialogue that meets the spiritual needs of patients. Institutions can support professional caregivers by providing resources for self-care and interdisciplinary teamwork that inspire spiritually competent practice. Social workers can take the lead by encouraging interdisciplinary team member collaboration and modeling the ongoing process of building spiritual competence as champions of *quality* spiritual care.

Achterberg, J., & Rothberg, D. (1996). Relationship as spiritual practice. *ReVision,19*(2), 2–8.

Ackley, B. J., Ladwig, G. B., & Makic, M. B. F. (2017). *Nursing diagnosis handbook: An evidence-based guide to planning* (11th ed.). St. Louis, MI: Elsevier.

Adams, G. (2006). [Review of the book *American spiritualities,* by C. L. Albanese]. *Nova Religio: The Journal of Alternative and Emergent Religions, 9*(3), 115–116. doi:10.1525/nr.2006.9.3.115.

Allamani, A. (2007). Suffering, choice, and freedom. *Substance Use & Misuse, 42,* 225–241. doi:10.1080/10826080601141966.

Almgren, G. R. (n.d.). *Palliative care with older adults. Section 3: Policy issues related to aging and palliative care.* Retrieved from www.cswe.org/File.aspx?id=24178.

Altilio, T., Gardia, G., & Otis-Green S. (2007). Social work practice in palliative and end-of-life care: A report from the Summit. *Journal of Social Work in End-of-Life & Palliative Care, 3*(4), 68–86. doi:10.1080/15524250802003513.

Anandarajah, G., & Hight, E. (2001). Spirituality and medical practice: Using the HOPE questions as a practical tool for spiritual assessment. *American Family Physician, 63,* 81–89.

Ando, M., Morita, T., Akechi, T., Ito, A., Tanaka, M., Ifuku, Y., & Nakayama, T. (2009). The efficacy of mindfulness-based meditation therapy on anxiety, depression, and spirituality in Japanese patients with cancer. *Journal of Palliative Medicine, 12*(12), 1091–1094. doi:10.1089=jpm.2009.0143.

Association for Spiritual, Ethical, and Religious Values in Counseling. (2009). *Competencies for addressing spiritual and religious issues in counseling.* Retrieved from www.aservic.org/wp-content/uploads/2010/04/Spiritual-Competencies-Printer-friendly.pdf.

Association of Professional Chaplains. (2000). *Association of Professional Chaplains code of ethics* [PDF document]. Retrieved from www.professionalchaplains.org/Files/professional_standards/professional_ethics/apc_code_of_ethics.pdf.

Association of Professional Chaplains. (2004a). *Common standards for professional chaplaincy* [PDF document]. Retrieved from www.professionalchaplains.org /files/professional_standards/common_standards/common_standards _professional_chaplaincy.pdf.

Association of Professional Chaplains. (2004b). *Common code of ethics for chaplains, pastoral counselors, pastoral educators and students* [PDF document]. Retrieved from www.professionalchaplains.org/files/professional_standards /common_standards/common_code_ethics.pdf.

Association of Professional Chaplains. (2015a). *Standards for board certified chaplains and associate certified chaplains* [DOC document]. Retrieved from http:// bcci.professionalchaplains.org/files/application_materials/general_standards .doc.

Association of Professional Chaplains. (2015b). *The standards of practice for professional chaplains in hospice and palliative care* [PDF document]. Retrieved from www.professionalchaplains.org/files/professional_standards/standards_of _practice/standards_of_practice_hospice_palliative_care.pdf.

Auty, S. (2005). Palliative care: Roles and perceptions. *International Journal of Palliative Nursing, 11*(2), 61.

Baggs, A., Wolf, C. P., Puig, A., and Fukuyama, M. (2009). *Integrating spiritual competencies into multicultural counseling* [PDF Document]. Retrieved from www.cherylpencewolf.com/images/documents/presentations/CPW-Spiritual Competencies-hndt-4-3-09.pdf.

Baker, N. (2005, December). [Review of the book *Working at relational depth in counselling and psychotherapy,* by D. Means & M. Cooper]. *Therapy Today, 16*(10), 55.

Balboni, T. A., Vanderwerker, L. C., Block, S. D., Paulk, M. E., Lathan, C. S., Peteet, J. R., & Prigerson, H. G. (2007). Religiousness and spiritual support among advanced cancer patients and associations with end-of-life treatment preferences and quality of life. *Journal of Clinical Oncology, 25*(4), 555–560. doi:10.1200/JCO.2006.07.9046.

Barber, C. (2012, December). Spirituality at the end-of-life: Where the HCA/AP can help. *British Journal of Healthcare Assistants, 6*(12), 596–599.

Belcher, A., & Griffiths, M. (2005). The spiritual care perspectives and practices of hospice nurses. *Journal of Hospice and Palliative Nursing, 7*(5), 271–279.

Bell, C. (2006). Paradigms behind (and before) the modern concept of religion. *History and Theory, 45,* 27–46.

Berzoff, J. (2008). It's never relative. [Review of the book *Relational theory and the practice of psychotherapy,* by P. A. Wachtel]. *Families in Society, 89,* 1–2. Retrieved from http://alliance1.org/sites/default/files/fis/BookReviewPDFs/3802_89_0 .pdf.

Bethel, J. C. (2004). Impact of social work spirituality courses on student attitudes, values, and spiritual wellness. *Journal of Religion & Spirituality in Social Work, 23*(4), 27–45. doi:10.1300/J377v23n04_03.

Blacker, S., Christ, G. H., & Lynch, S. (Eds.) (n.d.). *Charting the course for the future of social work in end-of-life and palliative care.* Retrieved from www.swhpn.org /monograph.pdf.

Blacker, S., & Deveau, C. (2010). Social work and interprofessional collaboration in palliative care. *Progress in Palliative Care, 18*(4), 237–243. doi:10.1179/09699 2610X12624290277141.

Bliss, J., & While, A. (2007). District nursing and social work: Palliative and continuing care delivery. *British Journal of Community Nursing, 12*(6), 268–272.

Branch, W. T. Jr., Torke, A., & Brown-Haithco, R. (2006). The importance of spirituality in African-Americans end-of-life experience. *Journal of General Internal Medicine, 21*(11), 1203–1205. doi:10.1 lll/j.1525-1497.2006.00572.x.

Bratton, D. (2005). *Spirituality: Faith and healthcare* [PowerPoint slides]. Retrieved from www.wdbydana.com/Spirituality.ppt.

Bregman, L. (2006). Spirituality: A glowing and useful term in search of a meaning. *Omega, 53*(1–2), 5–26.

Brennan, M. (2013). Four butterflies: End of life stories of transition and transformation. *Pastoral Psychology, 62,* 139–149. doi:10.1007/s11089-012-0477-5.

Briggs, M. K., & Rayle, A. D. (2005a). Incorporating spirituality into core counseling courses: Ideas for classroom application. *Counseling and Values, 50,* 63–75.

Briggs, M. K., & Rayle, A. D. (2005b). Spiritually and religiously sensitive counselors. In C. S. Cashwell & J. S. Young (Eds.), *Integrating spirituality and religion into counseling: A guide to competent practice* (pp. 85–104). Alexandria, VA: American Counseling Association.

Broughton, V. (2006). New SCM dictionary of Christian spirituality. *Reference Reviews, 20*(2), 16.

Buber, M. (1970). *I and thou.* (W. Kaufmann, Trans.). New York: Touchstone.

Buck, H. G., Overcash, J., & McMillan, S. C. (2009, November). The geriatric cancer experience at the end of life: Testing an adapted model. *Oncology Nursing Forum, 36*(6), 664–673.

Bullis, R. (1996). *Spirituality in social work practice.* Washington, DC: Taylor & Francis.

Bullock, K. (2011). The influence of culture on end-of-life decision making. *Journal of Social Work in End-of-Life & Palliative Care, 7,* 83–89. doi:10.1080 /15524256.2011.548048.

Büssing, A., Balzat, H. J., & Heusser, P. (2010). Spiritual needs of patients with chronic pain diseases and cancer—validation of the spiritual needs questionnaire. *European Journal of Medical Research, 15*(6), 266–273.

Butot, M. (2005). Reframing spirituality, reconceptualizing change: Possibilities for critical social work. *Critical Social Work, 6*(2). Retrieved from www1 .uwindsor.ca/criticalsocialwork/reframing-spirituality-reconceptualizing -change-possibilities-for-critical-social-work.

Bynum, J. P. W., Meara, E., Change, C. H., & Rhoads, J. M. (2016). *Our parents, ourselves: Health care for an aging population: A report of the Dartmouth Atlas Project* [PDF document]. Retrieved from www.dartmouthatlas.org/downloads /reports/Our_Parents_Ourselves_021716.pdf.

Byock, I. R. (1996). The nature of suffering and the nature of opportunity at the end of life. *Clinics in Geriatric Medicine, 12*(2), 237–252.

Callahan, A. M. (2008, October). *Spiritual caregiving: A research perspective.* Keynote address for the Lincoln Memorial University's Tri-State Social Work Roundtable in Harrogate, TN.

Callahan, A. M. (2009a, February). *Spiritual caregiving: A generalist perspective.* Workshop for the Social Workers of the Lakeway Area's Social Work Month Workshop in Morristown, TN.

Callahan, A. M. (2009b). Spiritually-sensitive care in hospice social work. *Journal of Social Work in End-of-Life and Palliative Care, 5*(3–4), *169–185.*

Callahan, A. M. (2011a, Fall). [Review of the book *The maintenance of life: Preventing social death through euthanasia talk and end-of-life care—lessons from the Netherlands*]. *Journal of Social Work Values and Ethics 8*(2). Available at www.socialworker.com/jswve/content/view/144/74/.

Callahan, A. M. (2011b, September/October). Spiritually sensitive hospice care. *Social Work Today, 11*(5), 25–27. Available at http://viewer.zmags.com/publication /b148f278#/b148f278/24.

Callahan, A. M. (2011c, October). *Relational spirituality: When professional helping enhances life meaning.* Workshop for the Fort Sanders Regional Medical Center Ethics Conference in Knoxville, TN.

Callahan, A. M. (2011d, October). *Teaching spiritual care: Resources and results.* Workshop presented for the North American Association of Christians in

Social Work's 61st Annual Convention in Pittsburgh, PA. Available at www
.nacsw.org/Publications/Proceedings2011/Proceedings2011.htm.

Callahan, A. M. (2012). A qualitative exploration of spiritually-sensitive hospice
care. *Journal of Social Service Research, 38*(2), 144–155.

Callahan, A. M. (2013). A relational model for spiritually-sensitive hospice care.
Journal of Social Work in End-of-Life and Palliative Care, 9(2–3), 158–179. doi:1
0.1080/15524256.2013.794051.

Callahan, A. M. (2015). Key concepts in spiritual care for hospice social workers:
How a multidisciplinary perspective can inform spiritual competence. *Social
Work & Christianity, 42*(1), 43–62. Available at www.nacsw.org/Publications
/SWC/SWC42_1.pdf.

Callahan, A. M. (2016, March). *Drawing from practice models to build spiritual
competence.* Workshop presented for the Social Work Hospice and Palliative
Care Network General Assembly in Chicago, IL. Available at https://c.ymcdn
.com/sites/swhpn.site-ym.com/resource/resmgr/SWHPN2016_Drawing
_from_Pract.pdf.

Callahan, A. M., Benner, K., & Helton, L. (2016). Facilitating spiritual competence through culturally responsive teaching. In M. Bart (Ed.), *Faculty focus
special report: Diversity and inclusion in the college classroom* (pp. 33-35). Madi-
son, WI: Magna Publications. Available at www.facultyfocus.com/free-reports
/diversity-and-inclusion-in-the-college-classroom/.

Campbell, C. L., & Ash, C. R. (2007). Keeping faith. *Journal of Hospice and Palliative Nursing, 9*(1), 31–41. doi:10.1177/0898010111418116.

Canda, E., & Furman, L. (1999). *Spiritual diversity in social work practice: The heart
of helping.* New York: Free Press.

Canda, E., & Furman, L. (2010). *Spiritual diversity in social work practice: The heart
of helping* (2nd ed.). New York: Free Press.

Canda, E. R. (1999). Spiritually sensitive social work: Key concepts and ideals. *Journal of Social Work, Theory, and Practice, 1*(1). Retrieved from www
.bemidjistate.edu/academics/publications/social_work_journal/issue01
/articles/canda.html.

Canda, E. R. (2005). Integrating religion and social work in dual degree programs.
Journal of Religion and Spirituality in Social Work, 24(1/2), 79–91.

Canning, D., Rosenberg, J. P., & Yates, P. (2007). Therapeutic relationships in spe-
cialist palliative care nursing practice. *International Journal of Palliative Nursing, 13*(5), 222–229.

Carroll, B. (2001). A phenomenological exploration of the nature of spirituality
and spiritual care. *Mortality, 6*(1), 81–98.

Carson, V. B., & Koenig, H. G. (2004). *Spiritual caregiving: Healthcare as a ministry*. Radnor, PA: Templeton Foundation Press.

Cassell, E. J. (1982). The nature of suffering and the goals of medicine. *New England Journal of Medicine, 306*(11), 639–645.

Cavendish, R., Konecny, L., Mitzeliotis, C., Russo, D., Luise, B., Lanza, M., Medefindt, J., & Bajo, M. A. (2003). Spiritual care activities of nurses using Nursing Interventions Classification (NIC) labels. *International Journal of Nursing Terminologies and Classifications, 14*(4), 113–124.

Center to Advance Palliative Care. (2012). Palliative care: What you should know [PDF document]. Retrieved from https://getpalliativecare.org/wp-content/uploads/2012/09/WhatYouShouldKnowHandoutRevised.pdf.

Centers for Medicare & Medicaid Services. (2012). *Cultural competency: A national health concern* [PDF document]. Retrieved from www.cms.gov/Outreach-and-Education/Medicare-Learning-NetworkMLN/MLNMattersArticles/downloads/SE0621.pdf.

Centers for Medicare & Medicaid Services. (n.d.). *Your Medicare Coverage: Hospice & respite care*. Retrieved from www.medicare.gov/coverage/hospice-and-respite-care.html.

Chatters, L. M., & Taylor, R. J. (2003). The role of social context in religion. *Journal of Religious Gerontology, 14*(2–3), 139–152. doi:10.1300/J078v14n02_04.

Chaturvedi, S. K. (2007). Spiritual issues at end of life. *Indian Journal of Palliative Care, 13*(2), 48–52.

Chochinov, H. M., & Cann, B. J. (2005). Interventions to enhance the spiritual aspects of dying. *Journal of Palliative Medicine, 8*(suppl. 1), 103–115.

Clark, L., Leedy, S., McDonald, L., Muller, B., Lamb, C., Mendez, T., . . . Schonwetter, R. (2007). Spirituality and job satisfaction among hospice interdisciplinary team members. *Journal of Palliative Medicine, 10*(6), 1321–1328. doi:10.1089/jpm.2007.0035.

Clausen, H., Kendall, M., Murray, S., Worth, A., Boyd, K., & Benton, F. (2005). Would palliative care patients benefit from social workers' retaining the traditional "casework" role rather than working as care managers? A prospective serial qualitative interview study. *British Journal of Social Work, 35*(2), 277–285. doi:10.1093/bjsw/bchl.

Collins, K. S., Furman, R., Hackman, R., Bender, K., & Bruce, E. A. (2007). Tending the soul: A teaching module for increasing student sensitivity to the spiritual needs of older adults. *Educational Gerontology, 33*, 707–722. doi:10.1080/03601270701364420.

Condition of Participation: Core Services, 42 C.F.R. § 418.64 (2010). Retrieved from www.gpo.gov/fdsys/pkg/CFR-2010-title42-vol3/xml/CFR-2010-title42 -vol3-part418-subpartC.xml.

Connor, S. R. (2007–2008). Development of hospice and palliative care in the United States. *Omega, 56*(1), 89–99.

Cooper, M. (2005). Therapists' experiences of relational depth: A qualitative interview study. *Counselling and Psychotherapy Research, 5*(2), 87–95. doi:10.1080 /14733140500211130.

Cooper, D., Aherne, M., & Pereira, J. (2010). The competencies required by professional hospice palliative care spiritual care providers. *Palliative Medicine, 13*(7), 869–875. doi:10.1089/jpm.2009.0429

Cornette, K. (2005). For whenever I am weak, I am strong . . . *International Journal of Palliative Nursing, 11*(3), 147–153.

Council on Social Work Education. (2008). *Education policy and accreditation standards.* Retrieved from www.cswe.org/File.aspx?id=41861

Council on Social Work Education. (2015a). *Education policy and accreditation standards.* Retrieved from www.cswe.org/File.aspx?id=81660

Council on Social Work Education. (2015b). *Religion and spirituality clearinghouse.* Retrieved from www.cswe.org/CentersInitiatives/CurriculumResources /50777.aspx.

Council on Social Work Education. (2015c). *Religion and spirituality educational resources.* Retrieved from www.cswe.org/CentersInitiatives/Curriculum Resources/50777/58508.aspx.

Coyle, B. R. (2001). Twelve myths of religion and psychiatry: Lessons for training psychiatrists in spiritually sensitive treatment. *Mental Health, Religion & Culture, 4*(2), 149–174. doi:10.1080/13674670110059541.

Creel, E. (2007). The meaning of spiritual nursing care for the ill individual with no religious affiliation. *International Journal for Human Caring, 11*(3), 16–21.

Crisp, B. R. (2011). If a holistic approach to social work requires acknowledgement of religion, what does this mean for social work education? *Social Work Education, 30*(6), 663–674.

Cunningham, M. (2012). *Integrating spirituality in clinical social work practice: Walking the labyrinth.* Upper Saddle River, NJ: Pearson Education.

Daaleman, T. P., Usher, B. M., Williams, S. W., Rawlings, J., & Hanson, L. C. (2008). An exploratory study of spiritual care at the end of life. *Annals of Family Medicine, 6*(5), 406–411.

Dahlin, C. (Ed.). (2013). *Clinical practice guidelines for quality palliative care* (3rd ed.). Pittsburg, PA: National Consensus Project for Quality Palliative Care.

Davis, D. E., Hook, J. N., & Worthington, E. L., Jr. (2008). Relational spirituality and forgiveness: The roles of attachment to God, religions coping, and viewing the transgression as a desecration. *Journal of Psychology and Christianity, 27*(4), 293–301.

Davis, D. E., Worthington, E. L., Jr., Hook, J. N., & Tongeren, D. R. V. (2009). The Dedication to the Sacred (DS) Scale: Adapting a marriage measure to study relational spirituality. *Journal of Psychology and Theology, 37*(4), 265–275.

Delgado-Guay, M. O., Hui, D., Parsons, H. A., Govan, K., De la Cruz, M., Tnorney, S., & Bruera, E. (2011). Spirituality, religiosity, and spiritual pain in advanced cancer patients. *Journal of Pain and Symptom Management, 41*(6), 986–994. doi:10.1016/j.jpainsymman.2010.09.017.

Derezotes, D. S. (2006). *Spiritually oriented social work practice.* Boston, MA: Pearson Education.

Dobratz, M. C. (2005). A comparative study of life-closing spirituality in home hospice patients. *Research and Theory for Nursing Practice: An International Journal, 19*(3), 243–256.

Doka, K. J. (2011). "Religion and spirituality: Assessment and intervention. *Journal of Social Work in End-of-Life and Palliative Care, 7*(1), 99–109.

Draper, P. (2011). *Spiritual care in healthcare: the state of the art* [PDF document]. Retrieved from www.viaa.nl/~/media/Files/Onderzoek/ZS/Diversen/20111104%20DraperP-handout.ashx.

Draper, P. (2012). An integrative review of spiritual assessment: Implications for nursing management. *Journal of Nursing Management, 20,* 970–980.

Driscoll, J. (2001). Spirituality and religion in end-of-life care. *Journal of Palliative Medicine, 4*(3), 333–335.

Dzul-Church, V., Cimino, J. W., Adler, S. R., Wong, P., & Anderson, W. G. (2010). "I'm sitting here by myself . . . ": Experiences of patients with serious illness at an urban public hospital. *Journal of Palliative Medicine, 13*(6), 695–701. doi:10.1089/jpm.2009.0352.

Edser, S. J., & May, C. (2007). Spiritual life after cancer: Connectedness and the will to meaning as an expression of self-help. *Journal of Psychosocial Oncology, 25*(1), 67–85. doi:10.1300/J077v25n01-04.

Edwards, A., Pang, N., Shiu, V., & Chan, C. (2010). The understanding of spirituality and the potential role of spiritual care in end-of-life and palliative care: A meta-study of qualitative research. *Palliative Medicine, 24*(8), 753–770. doi:10.1177/0269216310375860.

Egan, R., MacLeod, R., Jaye, C., McGee, R., Baxter, J., & Herbison, P. (2011). What is spirituality? Evidence from a New Zealand hospice study. *Mortality, 16*(4), 307–324. doi:10.1080/13576275.2011.613267.

Eilberg, R. A. (2006). Facing life and death: Spirituality in the end-of-life care. *Journal of Jewish Communal Service, 81*(3–4), 157–166.

Eisenhandler, S. A. (2005). "Religion is the finding thing": An evolving spirituality in late life. In H. R. Moody (Ed.), *Religion, spirituality, and aging: A social work perspective* (pp. 85–103). Binghamton, NY: Haworth. doi:10.1300/J083v45n01_06.

Elias, A. C. A., Giglio, J. S., & Pimenta, C. A. M. (2008). Analysis of the nature of spiritual pain in terminal patients and the resignification process through the relaxation, mental images and spirituality (RIME) intervention. *Revista Latino-Americana de Enfermagem, 16*(6), 959–965.

Ellison, C. G., & Lee, J. (2010). Spiritual struggles and psychological distress: Is there a dark side of religion. *Social Indicators Research, 98,* 501–516. doi:10.1007/s11205-009-9553-3.

Ellison, C. W. (1983). Spiritual well-being: Conceptualization and measurement. *Journal of Psychology and Theology, 11*(4), 330–340.

Emanuel, L. L., Alpert, H. R., Baldwin, D. C., & Emanuel, E. J. (2000). What terminally ill patients care about: Toward a validated construct of patients' perspectives. *Journal of Palliative Medicine, 3*(4), 419–431.

Exline, J. J., Prince-Paul, M., Root, B. L., & Peereboom, K. S. (2013). The spiritual struggle of anger toward god: A study with family members of hospice patients. *Journal of Palliative Medicine, 16*(4), 369–375. doi:10.1089/jpm.2012.0246.

Faver, C. A. (2004). Relational spirituality and social caregiving. *Social Work, 49*(2), 241–249.

Feller, C. P., & Cottone, R. R. (2003). The importance of empathy in the therapeutic alliance. *Journal of Humanistic Counseling, Education, and Development, 42,* 53–61.

Ferrell, B. (2011). Advancing the psychosocial care of patients with cancer at life's end: A global nursing response. *Oncology Nursing Forum, 38*(5), E335–E340.

Frank, R. K. (2009). Shared decision making and its role in end of life care. *British Journal of Nursing, 18*(10), 612–618.

Fukuyama, M. A., & Sevig, T. D. (1997). Spiritual issues in counseling: A new course. *Counselor Education & Supervision, 36*(3), 233–244.

Fukuyama, M. A. & Sevig, T. D. (1999). *Integrating spiritual issues into multicultural counseling.* Thousand Oaks, CA: Sage.

Furman, L. D., Benson, P. W., Canda, E. R., & Grimwood, C. (2004). A comparative international analysis of religion and spirituality in social work: A survey of UK and US social workers. *Social Work Education, 24*(8), 813–839.

Garces-Foley, K. (2006). Hospice and the politics of spirituality. *Omega, 53*(1–2), 117–136.

Gause, R., & Coholic, D. (2007). *Spiritually-influenced social work: A review of the literature.* Retrieved from www.stu.ca/~spirituality/gauselitreviewspiritualityand practice.pdf.

Gay, D. A., Lynxwiler, J. P., & Peek, C. W. (2001). The effects of switching on denominational subcultures. *Journal for the Scientific Study of Religion, 40*(3), 515–525.

Gert, B., Culver, C. M., & Clouser, K. D. (2006). *Bioethics: A systematic approach* (2nd ed.). New York: Oxford University Press.

Gijsberts, M. J., Echteld, M. A., van der Steen, J. T., Muller, M. T., Otten, R. H. J., Ribbe, M. W., & Deliens, L. (2011). Spirituality at the end of life: Conceptualization of measureable aspects—A systematic review. *Journal of Palliative Medicine, 14*(7), 852–863. doi:10.1089/jpm.2010.0356.

Gilligan, P., & Furness. S. (2006). The role of religion and spirituality in social work practice: Views and experiences of social workers and students. *British Journal of Social Work, 36,* 617–637.

Glasper, A. (2011). Can nurses enhance spiritual care in end-of-life settings? *British Journal of Nursing, 20*(5), 361–317.

Goddard, N. C. (1995). "Spirituality as integrative energy": A philosophical analysis as requisite precursor to holistic nursing practice. *Journal of Advanced Nursing, 22,* 808–815.

Goldberg, C., & Crespo, V. (2003). Suffering and personal agency. *International Journal of Psychotherapy, 8*(2), 85–93. doi:10.1080/1356908031000161273 4.

Goldsmith, J., Wittenberg-Lyles, E., Rodriguez, D., & Sanchez-Reilly, S. (2010). Interdisciplinary geriatric and palliative care team narratives: Collaboration practices and barriers. *Qualitative Health Research, 20*(1), 93–104.

Goldstein, E. D. (2007, October). Sacred moments: Implications on well-being and stress. *Journal of Clinical Psychology, 63*(10), 1001–19.

Gordon, T., & Mitchell, D. (2004). A competency model for the assessment and delivery of spiritual care. *Palliative Medicine, 18,* 646–651.

Graff, D. L., (2007). A study of baccalaureate social work students' beliefs about the inclusion of religious and spiritual content in social work. *Journal of Social Work Education, 43*(2), 243–256.

Grant, A. (2007). Spirituality, health and the complementary medicine practitioner. *Journal of the Australian Traditional-Medicine Society,13*(4), 207–209.

Grant, E., Murray, S. A., Kendall, M., Boyd, C., Tilley, S., & Ryan, D. (2004). Spiritual issues and needs: Perspectives from patients with advanced cancer and nonmalignant disease. A qualitative study. *Palliative and Supportive Care, 2,* 371–378. doi:10.10170S1478951504040490.

Gregory, J. E., & Gregory, R. J. (2004). The spiritual feather: An ecologically based celebration of life. *Palliative Medicine, 7,* 297–300.

Hall, T. W. (2004). Christian spirituality and mental health: A relational spirituality paradigm for empirical research. *Journal of Psychology and Christianity, 23*(1), 66–81.

Harrington, A. (2004). Hope rising out of despair: The spiritual journey of patients admitted to a hospice. In E. MacKinlay (Ed.), *Spirituality of later life: On humor and despair* (pp. 123–145). Binghamton, NY: Haworth.

Hay, D. (2000). Spirituality versus individualism: Why we should nurture relational consciousness. *International Journal of Children's Spirituality, 5*(1), 37–48.

Hebert, R., Zdaniuk, B., Schulz, R., & Scheier, M. (2009). Positive and negative religious coping and well-being in women with breast cancer. *Journal of Palliative Medicine, 12*(6), 537–545. doi:10.1089=jpm.2008.0250.

Henery, N. (2003a). Constructions of spirituality in contemporary nursing theory. *British Journal of Advanced Nursing, 42*(6), 550–557.

Henery, N. (2003b). The reality of visions: Contemporary theories of spirituality in social work. *British Journal of Social Work, 33*(8), 1105–1113.

Hermann, C. P. (2001). Spiritual needs of dying patients: A qualitative study. *Oncology Nursing Forum, 28*(1), 67–72.

Hermann, C. P. (2006). Development and testing of the spiritual needs inventory for patients near the end of life. *Oncology Nursing Forum, 33*(4), 737–744. doi:10.1188/06.ONF.737-744.

Hermann, C. P. (2007). The degree to which spiritual needs of patients near the end of life are met. *Oncology Nursing Forum, 34*(1), 70–78. doi:10.1188/07 .ONF.70-78.

Heyse-Moore, L. H. (1996). On spiritual pain in the dying. *Mortality, 1*(3), 297–315.

Hills, J., Paice, J., Cameron, J., & Shott, S. (2005). Spirituality and distress in palliative care consultation. *Journal of Palliative Medicine, 8*(4), 782–788.

Hodge, D. (2007a). The effect of spiritual characteristics on conceptualization
of spirituality and religion: A national study with a spiritually heterogeneous
sample. *Social Work & Christianity, 34*(1), 47–71.

Hodge, D. (2007b). The spiritual competence scale: A new instrument for assessing spiritual competence at the programmatic level. *Research on Social Work
Practice, 17*(2), 287–295.

Hodge, D. R. (2001). Spiritual assessment: A review of major qualitative methods
and a new framework for assessing spirituality. *Social Work, 46*(3), 203–214.

Hodge, D. R. (2003). *Spiritual assessment: Handbook for helping professionals.*
Botsford, CT: North American Association of Christians in Social Work Press.

Hodge, D. R. (2005a). Spirituality in social work education: A development and
discussion of goals that flow from the profession's ethical mandates. *Journal of
Social Work Education, 24*(1), 37–55.

Hodge, D. R. (2005b). Spiritual lifemaps: A client-centered pictorial instrument
for spiritual assessment, planning, and intervention. *Social Work, 50*(1), 77–87.

Hodge, D. R. (2007). The effect of spiritual characteristics on conceptualization
of spirituality and religion: A national study with a spiritually heterogeneous
sample. *Social Work & Christianity, 34*(1), 47–71.

Hodge, D. R. (2011). Using spiritual interventions in practice: Developing some
guidelines from evidence-based practice. *Social Work, 56*(2), 149–158.

Hodge, D. R., Baughman, L. M., & Cummings, J. A. (2006). Moving toward spiritual competency: Deconstructing religious stereotypes and spiritual prejudices
in social work literature. *Journal of Social Service Research, 32*(4), 211–231.

Hodge, D. R., & Bushfield, S. (2006). Developing spiritual competence in practice. *Journal of Ethnic & Cultural Diversity in Social Work, 15*(3–4), 101–127.
doi:10.1300/J051v15n03_05.

Hodge, D. R., & Horvath, V. E. (2011). Spiritual needs in health care settings: A
qualitative meta-synthesis of patients' perspectives. *Social Work, 56*(4), 306–316.

Hodge, D. R., & McGrew, C. C. (2005). Clarifying the distinctions and connections between spirituality and religion. *Social Work & Christianity, 32*(1), 1–21.

Holloway, M., Adamson, S., McSherry, W., & Swinton, J. (2011). *Spiritual care at
the end of life: A systematic review of the literature.* London, UK: Department
of Health.

Horton-Parker, R. J., & Fawcett, R. C. (2010). *Spirituality in counseling and psychotherapy: The face-spirit model.* Denver, CO: Love Publishing.

Horvath, A. O., Del Re, A. C., Flückiger, C., & Symonds, D. (2011). Alliance in individual psychotherapy. *Psychotherapy, 48*(1), 9–16. doi:10.1037/a0022186.

Hospice and Palliative Nurses Association. (2013, October). Patient/Family Teaching Sheet. *Spiritual distress* [PDF document]. Retrieved from www .stjosephhomehealth.org/documents/Spiritual-Distress-(English).pdf.

Hospice Foundation of America. (2005). *The dying process: A guide for caregivers* [Brochure]. Washington, DC: Author. Retrieved from www.optionsforeldercare .com/eldercarebooksandarticles/hospice_end_of_life_manual.pdf.

Hospice Foundation of America. (2011). *Addressing cultural diversity in hospice* [PDF document]. Retrieved from http://hospicefoundation.org/hfa/media /Files/hic_diversity_slides.pdf.

Hoyert, D. L. (2012, March). *75 years of morality in the United States, 1935–2010* (NCHS Data Brief, 88) [PDF document]. Hyattsville, MD: National Center for Health Statistics. Retrieved from www.cdc.gov/nchs/data/databriefs/db88 .pdf.

James, M. (2012). Where is the voice of social work in the multi disciplinary palliative care team? *Aotearoa New Zealand Social Work, 24*(2), 49–60.

Johnson, K., Elbert-Avila, K. J., & Tulsky, J. A. (2005). The influence of spiritual beliefs and practice on the treatment preferences of African Americans: A review of the literature. *Journal of American Geriatric Society, 53*(4), 711–719. doi:0002-8614/05.

Johnson, M. (2011). A randomized study of a novel Zen dialogue method for producing spiritual and well-being enhancement: Implications for end-of-life care. *Journal of Holistic Nursing, 29*(3), 201–210. doi:10.1177/0898010110391265.

Joint Commission. (2008). *Spiritual assessment.* Retrieved from www.joint commission.org/standards_information/jcfaqdetails.aspx?StandardsFaqId =290&ProgramId=47.

Joint Commission. (2016). *The Joint Commission: Over a century of quality and safety* [PDF document]. Retrieved from www.jointcommission.org/assets/1/6 /TJC_history_timeline_through_2015.pdf.

Kellehear, A. (2000). Spirituality and palliative care: A model of needs. *Palliative Medicine, 14*(2), 149–155.

Kim, S. C., Kim, S., & Boren, D. (2008). The quality of therapeutic alliance between patient and provider predicts general satisfaction. *Military Medicine, 173* (1), 85–90.

Kisvetrova, H., Kluger, M., & Kabelka, L. (2013). Spiritual support interventions in nursing care for patients suffering death anxiety in the final phase of life.

Knight, S. J., & von Gunten, C. (2004a). *How to assess spirituality.* Retrieved from http://endlink.lurie.northwestern.edu/religion_spirituality/part_one_when.cfm.

Knight, S. J. & von Gunten, C. (2004b). *Common needs and goals.* Retrieved from http://endoflife.northwestern.edu/religion_spirituality/part_two.pdf.

Knight, S. J., & von Gunten, C. (2004c). *Spiritual pain/spiritual suffering.* Retrieved from http://endoflife.northwestern.edu/religion_spirituality/part_three.pdf.

Knox, R. (2008). Clients' experiences of relational depth in person-centered counselling. *Counselling and Psychotherapy Research, 8*(3), 182–188. doi:10.1080/14733140802035005.

Knox, R., Murphy, D., Wiggins, S., & Cooper, M. (Eds.). (2013). *Relational depth: New perspectives and developments.* New York, NY: Palgrave Macmillan.

Kochanek, K. D., Murphy, S. L., Xu, J. Q., & Arias, E. (2014, December). *Mortality in the United States, 2013* (NCHS Data Brief, 178) [PDF document]. Hyattsville, MD: National Center for Health Statistics. Retrieved from www.cdc.gov/nchs/data/databriefs/db178.pdf.

Koenig, H. G. (2007). *Spirituality in patient care: Why, how, when, and what.* West Conshohocken, PA: Templeton Foundation Press.

Koenig, H. G. (2008). *Religion, spirituality, and health: Research and clinical applications* [PDF document]. Retrieved from: www.nacsw.org/Publications/Proceedings2008/KoenigHReligion.pdf.

Krieglstein, M. (2006). Spirituality and social work. *Dialogue and Universalism, 4–6,* 21–29.

Kulys, R., & Davis, M. (1986). An analysis of social services in hospice. *Social Work, 11*(6), 448–454.

Kulys, R., & Davis, M. (1987). Nurses and social workers: Rivals in the provision of social services? *Health & Social Work, 12*(2), 101–112.

Lamers, W. L. (2014). *Signs of approaching death.* Retrieved from http://hospicefoundation.org/End-of-Life-Support-and-Resources/Coping-with-Terminal-Illness/Signs-of-Approaching-Death.

Lamers, W. M. (2007). Reflections on "the last kiss." *Journal of Pain & Palliative Care Pharmacotherapy, 21*(3), 45–47. doi:10.1300/J354v21n03_08.

Langegard, U., & Ahlberg, K. (2009). Consolation in conjunction with incurable cancer. *Oncology Nursing Forum, 36*(2), E99–E106. doi:10.1188/09.ONF.E99-E106.

Larimore, W. L., Parker, M., & Crowther, M. (2002). Should clinicians incorporate positive spirituality into their practices? What does the evidence say? *Annals of Behavioral Medicine, 24*(1), 69–73.

Lawson, R. (2007). Home and hospital; hospice and palliative care: How the environment impacts the social work role. *Journal of Social Work in End-of-Life & Palliative Care, 3*(2), 3–17. doi:10.1300/J457v03n02_02.

Lee, M. Y., Ng, S., Leung, P. P. Y., & Chan, C. L. W. (2009). *Integrative body-mind-spirit social work: An empirically based approach to assessment and treatment.* New York: Oxford University Press.

Lukoff, D. (n.d.). *DSM-IV religious & spiritual problems* [PDF document]. Retrieved from www.spiritualcompetency.com/dsm4/dsmrsproblem.pdf.

MacConville, U. (2006). Mapping religion and spirituality in an Irish palliative care setting. *Omega, 53*(1–2), 137–152.

Mako, C., Galek, K., & Poppito, S. R. (2006). Spiritual pain among patients with advanced cancer in palliative care. *Journal of Palliative Medicine, 9*, 1106–1113.

Mathews, I. (2009). *Social work and spirituality.* Exeter, UK: Learning Matters.

Maugans, T. A. (1996). The SPIRITual history. *Archives of Family Medicine, 5*, 11–16.

McCormick, T. R. (2007). *Spirituality in medicine and healthcare* [PowerPoint slides]. Retrieved from http://courses.washington.edu/bh518/Spirituality Medicine UW-2007 (1).ppt.

McGrath, P., & Newell, C. (2004). The human connection: Study of spirituality and disability. *Journal of Religion, Disability & Health, 8*(1–2) 89–103.

McSherry, W., Cash, K., & Ross, L. (2004). Meaning of spirituality: Implications for nursing practice. *Journal of Clinical Nursing, 13*, 934–941.

Meador, K. G. (2006). Spirituality and care at the end of life. *Southern Medical Journal, 99*(10), 1184–1185.

Mearns, D. (1997). *Person-centred counselling training.* Thousand Oaks, CA: Sage Publications.

Mearns, D. (2003). *Developing person-centred counselling* (2nd ed.). London: Sage.

Mearns, D., & Cooper, M. (2005). *Working at relational depth in counselling and psychotherapy.* Thousand Oaks, CA: Sage.

Mearns, D., Thorne, B., & McLeod, J. (2013). *Person-centred counselling in action* (4th ed). Thousand Oaks, CA: Sage Publications.

Meier, D., & Beresford, L. (2008). Social workers advocate for a seat at palliative care table. *Journal of Palliative Medicine, 11*(1), 10–14. doi:10.1089/jpm.2008.9996.

Miller, D. K., Chibnall, J. T., Videen, S. D., & Duckro, P. N. (2005). Supportive-affective group for persons with life-threatening illness: Reducing spiritual, psychological, and death-related distress in dying patients. *Journal of Palliative Medicine, 8*(2), 333–343.

Milligan, S. (2011). Addressing the spiritual care needs of people near the end of life. *Nursing Standard, 26*(4), 47–56.

Millison, M. B. (1988). Spirituality and the caregiver: Developing an underutilized facet of care. *American Journal of Hospice Care, 5*(2), 37–44.

Mitchell, D. L., Bennett, M. J., & Manfrin-Ledet, L. (2006). Spiritual development of nursing students: Developing competence to provide spiritual care to patients at the end of life. *Journal of Nursing Education, 45*(9), 365–370.

Moadel, A., Morgan, C., Fatone, A., Grennan, J., Carter, J., Laruffa, G., ... Dutvher, J. (1999). Seeking meaning and hope: Self-reported spiritual and existential needs among an ethnically-diverse cancer patient population. *Psycho-oncology, 8,* 378–385.

Moberg, D. O. (2005). Research in spirituality, religion, and aging. *Journal of Gerontological Social Work, 45*(1–2), 11–40. doi:10.1300/J083v45n01_02.

Modesto, K. F., Weaver, A. J., & Flannelly, K. J. (2006). A systematic review of religious and spiritual research in social work. *Social Work & Christianity, 33*(1), 77–89.

Mok, E., & Chiu, P. C. (2004). Nurse-patient relationships in palliative care. *Journal of Advanced Nursing, 48*(5), 475–483.

Monroe, J., & DeLoach, R. J. (2004). Job satisfaction: How do social workers fare with other interdisciplinary team members in hospice settings? *Omega, 49*(4), 327–346.

Mount, B. M., Boston, P. H., & Cohen, S. R. (2007). Healing connections: On moving from suffering to a sense of well-being. *Journal of Pain and Symptom Management, 33*(4), 372–388.

Muehlbauer, P. M. (2013, March 5). Palliative care: Interdisciplinary team ensures comfort at the end of life. *Oncology Nursing Society Connect,* 28–32. Retrieved from http://connect.ons.org/issue/march-2013/up-front/palliative-care.

Murray, S. A., Kendall, M., Boyd, K., Worth, A., & Benton, T. F. (2004). Exploring the spiritual needs of people dying of lung cancer or heart failure: A prospective qualitative interview study of patients and their carers. *Palliative Medicine, 18,* 39–45.

Murray, S. A., Kendall, M., Grant, E., Boyd, K., Barclay, S., & Sheikh, A. (2007). Patterns of social, psychological, and spiritual decline toward the end of life in lung cancer and heart failure. *Journal of Pain and Symptom Management, 34*(4), 393–402. doi:10.1016/j.jpainsymman.2006.12.009.

Nakashima, M. (2007). Positive dying in later life: Spiritual resiliency among sixteen hospice patients. *Journal of Religion, Spirituality and Aging, 19*(2), 43–66.

Narayanasamy, A. (2007). Palliative care and spirituality. *Indian Journal of Palliative Care, 13*(2), 32–41, 43–66. doi:10.1300/J496v19n02_04.

National Association of Social Workers. (2001). *Indicators for the achievement of the NASW standards for cultural competence in social work practice* [Brochure]. Retrieved from www.naswdc.org/practice/standards/NAswculturalstandards.pdf.

National Association of Social Workers. (2004). *NASW standards for palliative & end of life care* [Brochure]. Retrieved from www.socialworkers.org/practice/bereavement/standards/standards0504New.pdf.

National Association of Social Workers. (2007). *Indicators for the achievement of the NASW standards for cultural competence in social work practice* [Brochure]. Retrieved from www.socialworkers.org/practice/standards/naswculturalstandards indicators2006.pdf.

National Association of Social Workers. (2008). *Code of ethics of the National Association of Social Workers*. Retrieved from www.socialworkers.org/pubs/code/code.asp.

National Association of Social Workers. (2015). *Indicators for the achievement of the NASW standards for cultural competence in social work practice* [Brochure]. Retrieved from www.socialworkers.org/practice/standards/PRA-BRO-253150-CC-Standards.pdf.

National Consensus Project for Quality Palliative Care. (2013). *Clinical practice guidelines for quality palliative care* (3rd ed.). Pittsburgh, PA: Author. Retrieved from www.nationalconsensusproject.org/Guidelines_Download2.aspx.

National Consensus Project for Quality Palliative Care. (2015). *Guidelines history*. Retrieved from www.nationalconsensusproject.org/DisplayPage.aspx?Title=Guidelines%20History

National Hospice and Palliative Care Organization. (n.d.a). *Medicare hospice conditions of participation spiritual caregiver*. Alexandria, VA: Author. Retrieved from www.nhpco.org/sites/default/files/public/regulatory/Spiritual_tip_sheet.pdf.

National Hospice and Palliative Care Organization. (n.d.b). *Inclusion and access*. Retrieved from www.nhpco.org/quality-10-components-quality-care/inclusion-and-access.

National Hospice and Palliative Care Organization (n.d.c). *Social work assessment tool (SWAT): Guidelines for use and completion.* Retrieved from www.nhpco .org/sites/default/files/public/nchpp/SWAT_Information_Booklet.pdf

National Hospice and Palliative Care Organization. (2007). *Offering spiritual support for family or friends* [Brochure]. N.p.: Author. Retrieved from www .caringinfo.org/files/public/brochures/faith_brochure.pdf.

National Hospice and Palliative Care Organization. (2014). *NHPCO facts and figures on hospice care in America.* Alexandria, VA: Author. Retrieved from www.nhpco.org/sites/default/files/public/Statistics_Research/2014_Facts _Figures.pdf.

National Hospice and Palliative Care Organization. (2015a). *History of hospice care.* Alexandria, VA: Author. Retrieved from www.nhpco.org/history-hospice -care.

National Hospice and Palliative Care Organization. (2015b). *The Medicare hospice benefit* [PDF document]. Retrieved from www.nhpco.org/sites/default/files /public/communications/Outreach/The_Medicare_Hospice_Benefit.pdf.

National Quality Forum. (2006). *A national framework and preferred practices for palliative and hospice care quality: A consensus report.* Washington, DC: Author. Retrieved from www.qualityforum.org/WorkArea/linkit.aspx?LinkIdentifier =id&ItemID=22041.

Nelson-Becker, H., & Canda, E. R. (2008). Spirituality, religion and aging research in social work: State of the art and future possibilities. *Journal of Religion, Spirituality & Aging, 20*(3), 177–193.

Nixon, A., & Narayanasamy, A. (2010). The spiritual needs of neuro-oncology patients from patients' perspective. *Journal of Clinical Nursing, 19,* 2259–2270. doi:10.1111/j.1365-2702.2009.03112.x.

Norcross, J. C. (Ed.). (2012). *Evidence-based therapy relationships* [PDF document]. Retrieved from www.nrepp.samhsa.gov/pdfs/Norcross_evidence-based_therapy _relationships.pdf.

North American Association of Christians in Social Work. (2008). *NACSW's mission and Christian identity.* Retrieved from www.nacsw.org/ChristianIdentity .htm.

Nuland, S. B. (1995). *How we die: Reflections of life's final chapter.* New York: Random House.

Ochs, C. (1986). *An ascent to joy: Transforming deadness of spirit.* Notre Dame, IN: University of Notre Dame Press.

Ochs, C. (1997). *Women and spirituality* (2nd ed.). Totowa, NJ: Rowman & Littlefield.

Okon, T. R. (2005) Spiritual, religious, and existential aspects of palliative care. *Journal of Palliative Medicine, 8*(2), 392–414.

Oliver, D. P., Washington, K. T., Wittenberg-Lyles, E., & Demiris, G. (2009). "They're part of the team": Participant evaluation of the active intervention. *Palliative Medicine, 23,* 549–555. doi:10.1177/0269216309105725.

Olthuis, J. (1994). Being-with: Toward a relational psychotherapy. *Journal of Psychology and Christianity, 13*(3), 217–231.

Open Society Foundations. (2015, October 11). *About us: History.* Retrieved from www.opensocietyfoundations.org/about/history.

Open Society Institute. (2004). *Transforming the culture of dying: The project on death in America October 1994 to December 2004* [PDF document]. Retrieved from www.opensocietyfoundations.org/sites/default/files/a_transforming.pdf.

Otis-Green, S. (2006). Spiritual palliative care. *Journal of Palliative Medicine, 9*(6), 1477–1478.

Pargament, K., Feuille, M. & Burdzy, D. (2011). The brief RCOPE: Current psychometric status of a short measure of religious coping. *Religions, 2,* 51–76. doi:10.3390/rel2010051.

Pargament, K., Smith, B. W., Koenig, H. G., & Perez, L. (1998). Patterns of positive and negative religious coping. *Journal for the Scientific Study of Religion, 37*(4), 710–724.

Pargament, K. I. (2007). *Spiritually integrated psychotherapy: Understanding and addressing the sacred.* New York: Guilford.

Pargament, K. I., & Ano, G. G. (2006). Spiritual resources and struggles in coping with medical illness. *Southern Medical Journal, 99*(10), 1161–1162.

Pargament, K. I., Koenig, H. G., Tarakeshwar, N., & Hahn, J. (2001). Religious struggle as a predictor of mortality among medically ill elderly patients: A 2-year longitudinal study. *Archive of Internal Medicine,161*(15), 1881–1885.

Pargament, K. I., Murray-Swank, N., Magyar, G., & Ano, G. (2005). Spiritual struggle: A phenomenon of interest to psychology and religion. In W. R. Miller and H. Delaney (Eds.), *Judeo-Christian perspectives on psychology: Human nature, motivation, and change* (pp. 245–268). Washington, DC: APA Press.

Parker-Oliver D., Bronstein L. R., & Kurzejeski L. (2005). Examining variables related to successful collaboration on the hospice team. *Health & Social Work, 30*(4), 279–86.

Parker-Oliver, D., & Peck, M. (2006). Inside the interdisciplinary team experiences of hospice social workers. *Journal of Social Work in End-of-Life & Palliative Care, 2*(3), 7–21. doi:10.1300/J457v02n03_03.

Payne, M. (2006). Identity politics in multiprofessional teams: Palliative care social work. *Journal of Social Work, 6,* 137–150. doi:10.1177/1468017306066741.

Payne, M. (2009). Developments in end-of-life and palliative care social work: International issues. *International Social Work, 52*(4), 513–524. doi:10.1177/0020872809104254.

Penman, J., Oliver, M., & Harrington, A. (2013). The relational model of spiritual engagement depicted by palliative care clients and caregivers. *International Journal of Nursing Practice, 19,* 39–46. doi:10.1111/ijn.12035.

Pesut, B. (2003). Developing spirituality in the curriculum: Worldviews, intrapersonal connectedness, interpersonal connectedness. *Nursing Education Perspectives, 24*(6), 290–294.

Pesut, B. (2008a). A conversation on diverse perspectives of spirituality in nursing literature. *Nursing Philosophy, 9,* 98–109.

Pesut, B. (2008b). A reply to "Spirituality and nursing: A reductionist approach" by John Paley. *Spirituality and Nursing, 9,* 131–137.

Pesut, B. (2008c). Spirituality and spiritual care in nursing fundamentals textbooks. *Journal of Nursing Education, 47*(4), 167–173. doi:10.3928/01484834-20080401-05.

Pesut, B., Fowler, M., Reimer-Kirkham, S., Taylor, E. J., & Sawatzky, R. (2009). Particularizing spirituality in points of tension: Enriching the discourse. *Nursing Inquiry, 16*(4), 337–346.

Pesut, B., Sinclair, S., Fitchett, G., Greg, M., & Koss, S. E. (2016). Health care chaplaincy: A scoping review of the evidence 2009–2014. *Journal of Health Care Chaplaincy, 22,* 67–84. doi:10.1080/08854726.2015.1133185.

Peteet, J. R., & Balboni, M. J. (2013). Spirituality and religion in oncology. *CA: A Cancer Journal for Clinicians, 63,* 280–289. doi:10.1002/caac.21187.

Pevey, C. F., Jones, T. J., & Yarber, A. (2009). How religion comforts the dying: A qualitative inquiry. *Omega, 58*(1), 41–59. doi:10.2190/OM.58.1.c.

Pike, J. (2011). *Spirituality in nursing: A systematic review of the literature from 2006–10, 20*(12), 743–749.

Priebe, S., & McCabe, R. (2008). Therapeutic relationships in psychiatry: The basis of therapy or therapy in itself? *International Review of Psychiatry, 20*(6), 521–526. doi:10.1080/09540260802565257.

Prince-Paul, M. (2008). Understanding the meaning of social well-being at the end of life. *Oncology Nursing Forum, 35*(3), 365–371. doi:10.1188/08 .ONF.365-371.

Puchalski, C., Ferrel, B., Virani, R., Otis-Green, S., Baird, P., Bull, J., . . . Sulmasy, D. (2009). Improving the quality of spiritual care as a dimension of palliative care: The report of the consensus conference. *Journal of Palliative Medicine, 12*(10), 885–904. doi:10.1089/jpm.2009.0142.

Puchalski, C. M. (2001). The role of spirituality in health care. *Baylor University Medical Center Proceedings, 14*(4), 352–357.

Puchalski, C. M. (2006). *A time for listening and caring: Spirituality and the care of the chronically ill and dying.* New York: Oxford University Press.

Puchalski, C. M. (2008a). Addressing the spiritual needs of patients. In P. Angelos (Ed.), *Ethical issues in cancer patient care* (2nd ed., pp. 79–91). New York: Springer Science+Business. doi:10.1007/978-0-387-73639-6_6.

Puchalski, C. M. (2008b). Honoring the sacred in medicine: Spirituality as an essential element of patient-centered care. *Journal of Medicine and the Person, 6*(3), 113–117. doi:10.2190/OM.56.1.d.

Puchalski, C. M. (2008c). Spirituality and the care of patients at the end-of-life: An essential component of care. *Omega, 56*(1), 33–46. doi:10.2190/OM.56.1.d.

Puchalski, C. M. (2013). Integrating spirituality into patient care: An essential element of person-centered care. *Polish Archives of Internal Medicine, 123*(9), 491–497.

Puchalski, C. M., Lunsford, B., Harris, M. H., & Miller, T. (2006). Interdisciplinary spiritual care for seriously ill and dying patients: A collaborative model. *Cancer Journal, 12*(5), 389–416.

Puchalski, C. M. & Romer, A. L. (2000). Taking a spiritual history allows clinicians to understand patients more fully. *Journal of Palliative Medicine, 3*(1), 129–137.

Raghavan, M., Smith, A. K., & Arnold, R. M. (2010). African Americans and end-of-life care #204. *Journal of Palliative Medicine, 13*(11), 1382–1383. doi:10.1089 /jpm.2010.9762.

Reese, D. (2011a). Spirituality and social work practice in palliative care. In Terry Altilio & Shirley Otis-Green (Eds.). *Oxford textbook of palliative social work* (pp. 201–214). New York: Oxford University Press.

Reese, D., & Brown, D. (1997). Psychosocial and spiritual care in hospice: Differences between nursing, social work, and clergy. *Hospice Journal, 12*(1), 29–41.

Reese, D., Raymer, M., Orloff, S., Gerbino, S., Valade, R., Dawson, S., ... Huber, R. (2006). The Social Work Assessment Tool (SWAT). *Journal of Social Work in End-of-Life and Palliative Care, 2*(2), 65–95.

Reese, D. J. (2001). Addressing spirituality in hospice: Current practices and a proposed role for transpersonal social work. In E. R. Canda & E. D. Smith (Eds.), *Transpersonal perspectives on spirituality in social work* (pp. 135–161). Binghamton, NY: Haworth.

Reese, D. J. (2011b). Interdisciplinary perceptions of the social work role in hospice: Building upon the classic Kulys and Davis study. *Journal of Social Work in End-of-Life & Palliative Care, 7,* 383–406. doi:10.1080/15524256.2011.623474.

Reese, D. J. (2013). Hospice social work. *End-of-life care: A series.* New York: Columbia University Press.

Reese, D. J., Chan, C. W., Chan, W. C. H., & Wiersgalla, D. (2010). Cross-national comparison of Hong Kong and U.S. student beliefs and preferences in end-of-life care: Implications for social work education and hospice practice. *Journal of Social Work in End-of-Life & Palliative Care, 6,* 205–235. doi:10.1080/15524256.2010.529021.

Reese D. J., & Raymer M. (2004). Relationships between social work involvement and hospice outcomes: Results of the National Hospice Social Work Survey. *Social Work, 49*(3), 415–422.

Reith, M., & Payne, M. (2009). *Social work in end-of-life and palliative care.* Chicago, IL: Lyceum.

Rice, S., & McAuliffe, D. (2009). Ethics of the spirit: Comparing ethical views and usages of spiritually influenced interventions. *Australian Social Work, 62*(3), 403–420.

Rogers, C. R. (2007). The necessary and sufficient conditions of therapeutic personality change. *Psychotherapy: Theory, Research, Training, 44*(3), 240–248.

Rogers, S. A. (2007). Where the moment meets the transcendent: Using the process as a spiritual intervention in object relations psychotherapy. *Journal of Psychology and Christianity, 26*(2), 151–158.

Sandage, S. J., & Shults, F. L. (2007). Relational spirituality and transformation: A relational integration model. *Journal of Psychology and Christianity, 26*(3), 261–269.

Sandage, S. J., & Williamson, I. (2010). Relational spirituality and dispositional forgiveness: A structural equations model. *Journal of Psychology and Theology, 38*(4), 255–266.

Sanger, M. (2010). The four-quadrant framework for addressing spiritual and religious issues in social work. *Journal of Baccalaureate Social Work, 15*(1), 91–103.

Saunders, C. (1988). Spiritual pain. *Journal of Palliative Care, 4*(3), 30.

Saunders, S. (2001). Pretreatment correlates of the therapeutic bond. *Journal of Clinical Psychology, 57*(12), 1339–1352.

Saunders, C. (2005). *Watch with me: Inspiration for a life in hospice care.* Bailrigg, UK: Observatory Publications.

Schneiders, S. M. (2003). Religion vs. spirituality: A contemporary conundrum. *Spiritus, 3,* 163–185.

Senreich, E. (2013). An inclusive definition of social work education. *Journal of Social Work Education, 49*(4), 548–563. doi:10.1080/10437797.2013.812460.

Sessanna, L., Finnell, D. S., Underhill, M., Chang, Y. P., & Peng, H. L. (2011). Measures assessing spirituality as more than religiosity: A methodological review of nursing and health-related literature. *Journal of Advanced Nursing, 67*(8), 1677–1694. doi:10.1111/j.1365-2648.2010.05596.x.

Seyfried, S. F. (2007). Creating a diverse spirituality community: Reflections from a spirituality and social work practice class. *Journal of Ethnic & Cultural Diversity in Social Work, 16*(3–4), 159–167. doi:10.1300/J051vl6n03_13.

Sheldon, J. E. (2000). Spirituality as part of nursing. *Journal of Hospice and Palliative Nursing, 2*(3) 101–108.

Sherburne, C. (2008). Spirituality: The beauty secret of aging. *LLI Review, 3,* 102–108.

Sheridan, M. (2009). Ethical issues in the use of spiritually based interventions in social work practice: What are we doing and why. *Social Thought, 28*(1–2), 99–126.

Simpson, D. B., Newman, J. L., & Fuqua, D. R. (2008). Understanding the role of relational factors in Christian spirituality. *Journal of Psychology and Theology, 36*(2), 124–134.

Sinclair, S., Pereira, J., & Raffin, S. (2006). A thematic review of the spirituality literature within palliative care. *Journal of Palliative Medicine, 9*(2), 464–479.

Skovholt, T. M. (2005). The cycle of caring: A model of expertise in the helping professions. *Journal of Mental Health Counseling, 27*(1), 82–93.

Sloan, R. P., Bagiella, E., VandeCreek, L., Hover, M., Casalone, C., Hirsch, T. J., . . . Poulos, P. (2000). Should physicians prescribe religious activities? *New England Journal of Medicine, 342*(25), 1913–1916.

Smith, A. R. (2006). Using the synergy model to provide spiritual nursing care in critical care settings. *Critical Care Nurse, 26*(4), 41–47.

Smith, A. R., DeSanto-Madeya, S., Perez, J. E., Tracy, E. F., DeCristofaro, S., Norris, R. L., & Mukkamala, S. L. (2012). How women with advanced cancer pray: A report from two focus groups. *Oncology Nursing Forum, 39*(3), E310–E316.

Smith-Stoner, M. (2007). End-of-life preferences for atheists. *Journal of Palliative Medicine, 10*(4), 923–928. doi:10.1089/jpm.2006.0197.

Social Work Hospice and Palliative Care Network. (2013). *Our story*. Retrieved from www.swhpn.org/our-story.

Society for Spirituality and Social Work. (n.d.). *Spiritual competencies*. Retrieved from http://societyforspiritualityandsocialwork.com/pdfs/SpiritualCompetencies[1].pdf.

Sperry, L. (2010). Psychotherapy sensitive to spiritual issues: A postmaterialist psychology perspective and developmental approach. *Psychology of Religion and Spirituality, 2*(1), 46–56. doi:I 0.10.37/a00 8549.

Sperry, L., & Miller, L. (2010). *Spirituality in clinical practice: Theory and practice of spiritually oriented psychotherapy* (2nd ed.). New York: Routledge.

Stanworth, R. (2006). When spiritual horizons beckon: Recognizing ultimate meaning at the end of life. *Omega, 53*(1–2), 27–36.

Staude, J. (2005). Autobiography as a spiritual practice. *Journal of Gerontological Social Work, 45*(3), 249–269.

Stephenson, P., Draucker, C. B., and Martsolf, D. S. (2003). The experience of spirituality in the lives of hospice patients. *Journal of Hospice and Palliative Nursing, 5*(1), 51–58.

Stern, J., & James, S. (2006). Every person matters: Enabling spirituality education for nurses. *Journal of Clinical Nursing, 15*, 897–904. doi:10.1111/j.1365-2702.2006.01663.x.

Stirling, I. (2007). The provision of spiritual care in a hospice: Moving towards a multi-disciplinary perspective. *Scottish Journal of Healthcare Chaplaincy, 10*(2), 21–27.

Sulmasy, D. P. (2002). A biopsychosocial-spiritual model for the care of patients at the end of life. *Gerontologist, 42*, 24–33.

Sulmasy, D. P. (2009). Spirituality, religion, and clinical care. *Chest, 135*, 1634–1642. doi 10.1378/chest.08-2241.

Svare, G. M., Jay, S., Bruce, E., & Owens-Kane, S. (2003). Going below the tip of the iceberg: Social work, religion, and spirituality. *Social Thought, 22*(4), 19–35. doi:10.1300/J131v22n04_03.

Swinton, J., & Pattison, S. (2010). Moving beyond clarity: Towards a thin, vague, and useful understanding of spirituality in nursing care. *Nursing Philosophy, 11,* 226–237.

Takahashi, M., & Ide, S. (2003). Implicit theories of spirituality across three generations: A cross-cultural comparison in the U.S. and Japan. *Journal of Religious Gerontology, 15*(4), 15–38. doi:10.1300/J078v15n04_03.

Tan, H. M., Braunack-Mayer, A., & Beilby, J. (2005). The impact of the hospice environment on patient spiritual expression. *Oncology Nursing Forum, 32*(5), 1049–1055.

Taylor, E. J. (2007). *What do I say? Talking with patients about spirituality.* West Conshohocken, PA: Templeton Foundation Press.

Taylor, E. J., & Mamier, I. (2004). Spiritual care nursing: What cancer patients and family caregivers want. *Journal of Advanced Nursing, 49*(3), 260-267.

Thune-Boyle, I. C., Stygall, J. A., Keshtgar, M. R., & Newman, S. P. (2006). Do religious/spiritual coping strategies affect illness adjustment in patients with cancer? A systematic review of the literature. *Social Science & Medicine, 63,* 151–164. doi:10.1016/j.socscimed.2005.11.055.

Touhy, T. A., Brown, C., & Smith, C. J. (2005). Spiritual caring: End of life in a nursing home. *Journal of Gerontological Nursing, 31*(9), 27–35.

Tuck, I., Johnson, S. C., Kuznetsova, M. I., McCrocklin, C., Baxter, M., & Bennington, L. K. (2012). Sacred healing stories told at the end of life. *Journal of Holistic Nursing, 30*(2), 69–80. doi:10.1177/0898010111418116.

United States Centers for Disease Control and Prevention. (2015, February 6). *Deaths: Final data for 2013* [PDF document]. Retrieved from www.cdc.gov /nchs/data/nvsr/nvsr64/nvsr64_02.pdf.

University of Alabama. (n.d.). *4.2. Spiritual distress: Fostering transcendence at life's end* [PDF document]. Retrieved from http://services.medicine.uab.edu/public documents/palliativecare/resident/spiritual/palliative_response_4_1-2.pdf.

Vachon, M., Fillion, L., & Achille, M. (2009). A conceptual analysis of spirituality at the end of life. *Journal of Palliative Medicine, 12*(1), 53–59. doi:10.1089/jpm.2008.0189.

Vallurupalli, M., Lauderdale, K., Balboni, M. J., Phelps, A. C., Block, S. D., Ng, A. K., . . . Balboni, T. A. (2011). The role of spirituality and religious coping in the quality of life of patients with advanced cancer receiving palliative radiation therapy. *Journal of Supportive Oncology, 20*(10), 1–7. doi:10.1016/j .suponc.2011.09.003.

Van der Steen, J. T., Gijsberts, M. H. E., Echteld, M. A., Muller, M. T., Ribbe, M. W., & Deliens, L. (2009). Defining spirituality at the end of life. *Journal of Palliative Medicine, 12*(8), 677. doi:10.1089/jpm.2009.0103.

Van Hook, M. P., & Rivera, J. O. (2004). Coping with difficult life transitions by older adults: The role of religion. *Social Work & Christianity, 31*(3), 233–253.

Walter, T. (2002). Spirituality in palliative care: Opportunity or burden? *Palliative Medicine, 16*(2), 133–139.

Ward, T. (2005) Introduction: "I'm really not religious": Spirituality in the twenty-first century. *Sewanee Theological Review, 48*(2), 139–140.

Warwick, L. L. (2001). Self-in-relation theory and women's religious identity in therapy. In E. Kaschak (Ed.), *The invisible alliance: Psyche and spiritual in feminist therapy* (pp. 121–131). Binghamton, NY: Haworth.

Wasner, M., Longaker, C., Fegg, M. J., & Borasio, G. D. (2005). Effects of spiritual care training for palliative care professionals. *Journal of Palliative Medicine, 19*(2), 99–104. doi:10.1191/0269216305pm995oa.

Weatherby, G. A. (2002). [Review of the book *American spiritualities: A reader*, by C. L. Albanese]. *Sociology of Religion, 63*, 4. doi:10.2307/3712306.

Whitfield, C. L. (1984). Stress management and spirituality during recovery: A transpersonal approach. Part 1: Becoming. *Alcoholism Treatment Quarterly, 1*(1), 3–54.

Winkelman, W. D., Lauderdale, K., Balboni, M. J., Phelps, A. C., Peteet, J. R., Block, S. D., . . . Balboni, T. A. (2011). The relationship of spiritual concerns to the quality of life of advanced cancer patients: Preliminary findings. *Journal of Palliative Medicine, 14*(9), 1022–1028. doi:10.1089/jpm.2010.0536.

Wintz, S., & Cooper, E. (2003). *Learning module: Cultural and spiritual sensitivity* [PDF document]. Retrieved from www.healthcarechaplaincy.org /userimages/Cultural_Spiritual_Sensitivity_Learning_ percent20Module percent 207-10-09.pdf.

Wintz, S. K. (2004). The chaplain's path in cultural and spiritual sensitivity: A response to Anderson, Fukuyama, and Sevig. In R. G. Anderson & M. A. Fukuyama (Eds.), *Ministry in the spiritual and cultural diversity of health care: Increasing competency of chaplains* (pp. 71–82). Binghamton, NY: Haworth. doi:10.1300/J080v13n02_06.

Wittenberg-Lyles, E., Parker-Oliver, D., Demiris, G., Baldwin, P., & Regehr, K. (2008). Communication dynamics in hospice teams: Understanding the role of the chaplain in interdisciplinary team collaboration. *Journal of Palliative Medicine, 11*(10), 1330–1335. doi:10.1089/jpm.2008.0165.

Wong, Y. R., & Vinsky, J. (2009). Speaking from the margins: A critical reflection on the "spiritual-but-not-religious" discourse in social work. *British Journal of Social Work, 39,* 1343–1359. doi:10.1093/bjsw/bcn032.

Wright, M. C. (2002). The essence of spiritual care: A phenomenological enquiry. *Palliative Medicine, 16*(2), 125–132.

Wynne, L. (2013, September 11). Spiritual care at the end of life. *Nursing Standard, 28*(2), 41–45.

Yalom, I. D. (1995). *The theory and practice of group psychotherapy.* New York: Basic.

Yang, W., Staps, T., & Hijmans, E. (2010). Existential crisis and the awareness of dying: The role of meaning and spirituality. *Omega, 61*(1), 53–69. doi:10.2190/OM.61.1.c.

Yardley, S. J., Walshe, C. E., & Parr, A. (2009). Improving training in spiritual care: A qualitative study exploring patient perceptions of professional educational requirements. *Palliative Medicine, 23,* 601–607. doi:10.1177/0269216309105726.

Zapf, M. K. (2008). Transforming social work's understanding of person and environment: Spirituality and the "common ground." *Social Thought, 27*(1–2), 171–181. doi:10.1080/15426430802114200.